Group

The International Library of Group Analysis

Edited by Malcolm Pines, Institute of Group Analysis, London

The aim of this series is to represent innovative work in group psychotherapy, particularly but not exclusively group analysis. Group analysis, taught and practised widely in Europe, has developed from the work of S.H. Foulkes.

Other titles in the series

Circular Reflections
Selected Papers on Group Analysis and Psychoanalysis
Malcolm Pines
International Library of Group Analysis 1
ISBN 1 85302 492 9 paperback
ISBN 1 85302 493 7 hardback

Attachment and Interaction
Mario Marrone with a contribution by Nicola Diamond
International Library of Group Analysis 3
ISBN 1 85302 587 9 hardback
ISBN 1 85302 586 0 paperback

Self Experiences in Group
Intersubjective and Self Psychological Pathways to Human Understanding
Edited by Irene Harwood and Malcolm Pines
International Library of Group Analysis 4
ISBN 1 85302 596 8 hardback
ISBN 1 85302 610 7 paperback

Taking the Group Seriously
Towards a Post-Foulkesian Group Analytic Theory
Farhad Dalal
International Library of Group Analysis 5
ISBN 1 85203 642 5 paperback

Active Analytic Group Therapy for Adolescents
John Evans
International Library of Group Analysis 6
ISBN 1 85302 616 6 paperback
ISBN 1 85302 617 4 hardback

The Group Context
Sheila Thompson
International Library of Group Analysis 7
ISBN 1 85302 657 3 paperback

INTERNATIONAL LIBRARY OF GROUP ANALYSIS 8

Group

Claudio Neri

Preface by Parthenope Bion Talamo

Foreword by Malcolm Pines

Jessica Kingsley Publishers
London and Philadelphia

First published in Italian in 1995 under the title of *Gruppo* by Edizione Borla s.r.l., Roma.

First published in English in the United Kingdom in 1998 by
Jessica Kingsley Publishers Ltd
116 Pentonville Road
London N1 9JB, England
and
325 Chestnut Street
Philadelphia, PA 19106, USA

Library of Congress Cataloging in Publication Data
A CIP catalogue record for this book is available from the
Library of Congress

British Library Cataloguing in Publication Data
A CIP catalogue record for this book is available from the
British Library

ISBN 1 85302 418 X

Printed and Bound in Great Britain by
Athenaeum Press, Gateshead, Tyne and Wear

Contents

Acknowledgements

I feel extremely gratified by this English language edition of *Group*. Group psychotherapy had its origins in Great Britain and the United States and a fine tradition is being followed up by colleagues in these countries. My hope is that the translation of *Group* will contribute to and increase my scientific collaboration with them.

Another reason for my pleasure at the publication of this book is my personal links with these two countries since I had my first medical experiences as an intern in a London hospital and carried out a part of my psychiatric training in New York.

My sincere thanks go to R. Hinshelwood and M. Pines whose generous and enthusiastic support made possible the translation of this book.

I should also like to thank C. Trollope who translated the text with discernment and professional ability. Other colleagues, namely L. Baglione, G.S. Gunzi Danile, V. Coata Sternberg, G. Nebbiosi and M. Paterno, read the translation and offered much appreciated advice.

This book is the result of many years' work together with colleagues at the Centre for Psychoanalytical Research, 'Il Pollaiolo', co-researchers of the Department of Theory and Technique of Group Dynamics of the Faculty of Psychology of the 'La Sapienza' University, and the staff of the Department of Mental Health RMB U.O.T. 7. A. My heartfelt thanks to all of them.

My special thanks and appreciation go to those people whose nearness was of special value to me: Francesco Corrao who shares with me his passion for psychoanalysis and for group analysis, Antonio Correale, Nino Dazzi, Eugenio Gaburri, Stefania Marinelli, Romolo Petrini, Roberto Pomar, who are my friends in life and at work, Alessandro Bruni, Giorgio Corrente, Maria Bruna Dorliguzzo, with whom I discussed in detail many subjects dealt with in this book.

People who made a significant contribution to the preparation of the book were Marco Bernabei, Luisa De Bellis, Silvia Contorni, Fortunata Gatti, Luciana Marinese, Marco Longo and Gianni Nebbiosi, who read the typescript and made valuable suggestions; Paola Fadda who compiled the analytic index; and Parthenope Bion Talamo who wrote the preface. Affectionate thanks to them all.

Special thanks to Vincenzo d'Agostino for advice on the graphic and editorial form, Antonio Verdolin for revising the text, and Tiziana Iarossi and Laura Salvaggi for competently polishing and redrafting the material.

Preface

The elegantly succinct title of this book, *Group*, by Claudio Neri reveals one of its most important ideas, one of its fundamental characteristics, but one which is never directly explained as such. Here Neri is speaking of a certain type of human aggregation, so common in every type of society that we may suppose that it is a characteristic of the species, so that his universe of discourse is not limited to the narrow spaces of artificially formed research groups, but refers to all human groups, without the distinction between group and mass becoming blurred. This choice, which widens the discussion on groups and takes it beyond the limits of psychopathology or professional training also explains why the book has a series of characteristics which make it particularly pleasurable and enriching to read, such as the frequent use of examples taken from world literature, especially from the east, to illustrate theoretical points, which gain much from being thus situated in their natural humus.

Another fundamental characteristic of this book is the way in which it can be said to be a 'group' itself, in two different senses. Neri does not limit himself to placing his subject within the 'human condition', but also carries on a dialogue with colleagues of the past and the present; it is not a 'dutiful' (and therefore perhaps also boring?) series of references to the more or less sacred scriptures of authors, well known or not, who have already written on this subject, but a lively conversation at a distance, which weighs up what has been said by the one and compares it with similar – or contrasting – concepts of the other. Neri's own argument gains depth and richness from the toing and froing between other authors, without any pedantic heaviness, leaving the reader with the image of the author as belonging to an ideal group of scholars. But there is another sense in which the book itself becomes a group; not in the contents, but in the way in which these are bound together. The structure of the text refers back to the network – or rather networks – which develop on many levels within every group. We can take the various parts of the book, which are necessarily printed and joined together one after the other, as though they belonged in reality to a building with many floors; one can walk around on a single floor, or one can take the lifts. In the reality of the book these 'lifts' are the copious mentions and references to coming chapters, the task of which is to amplify ideas the author has earlier introduced only briefly, or to counsel the reader, who has by then come to grips with a denser and harder theoretical passage, to take up again for a moment the discussion at the point at which a new concept has been introduced for the first time.

Besides these references, the book has been endowed with two other features which make reading considerably easier; the first of these are the panels in which some concepts are treated in very short historical/critical notes, which are a decided improvement on the usual footnotes, because they can be read or skipped after a very rapid glance to decide whether the reader needs the information contained in them at that particular stage. These panels are in some way analogous to the 'digressions' which may be found in a conversation between a group of friends, and do not distract attention from the main text. The excellent glossary is a further tool, extremely useful again as a mental place to return to every now and then to clarify the most thorny points of the text. Despite the fact that this is a decidedly user-friendly book, it is nevertheless not easy on the conceptual level. When Claudio Neri very kindly asked me to write this short preface I felt not only honoured, but also distinctly worried, because of the multitude and density of the arguments – even though relieved by the technique of writing and the physical structure of the text – and because of the complex way in which they are linked together. I do not think it is possible to do justice to a book of this sort in a few words, so I shall limit myself to giving an indication of what I think is the problem which the author's thoughts are seeking to elucidate, and I shall leave to the reader the pleasure of discovering the details of the heuristic instruments which Neri, equipped with all his human and professional experience, has decided to use in this considerable task.

Neri introduces two series of concepts (field, semiosphere, protomental system on the one hand, and fraternal community, commuting, trans-personal diffusion, and disposition in the shape of a star on the other) which are intended to describe and throw light on everything pre-verbal, non-verbal and beyond the verbal which can be met when the group is studied as an entity and when something has to be said about the group which gives a bird's-eye view and does not just stay on the ground inside the group. (That is to say, a metadiscourse which can be limited to the theoretical realm or can (also) be therapeutical.) The first series of concepts pertains to theories on the state of the group, on its conditions, while the second refers to the way in which the group behaves when certain conditions are fulfilled. These two levels are constantly interwoven, both seeking, in different ways, for the answer to the problem of what non-verbal or extra-verbal phenomena occur in human communication, and how they occur in practice. The great problem of extra-verbal communication can be intuitively sensed principally as lying behind the concept of 'field': the 'field' seems to be introduced so as to be able to speak of this problem in a different way from the American theory of micro-communication (facial mimicry, posture etc.) but there still remain difficulties in knowing how projective identifications are 'conveyed' from one person to another, how they are communicated.

In this book Neri has tried to show how all this can be thought about, how adequate tools for our requirements can be acquired, and what sort of use to make of them. One of the difficulties that he certainly came across when setting about this task is a cultural fact: human beings in general tend to speak, and psychoanalysis in particular has valued (and possibly overvalued) speech, not considering it simply as the one effective therapeutic means – and this is one of the basic concepts of psychoanalysis, part of its structure and definition – but surreptitiously taking as being 'good' or 'valid' principally verbal communication, to the detriment of non-verbal. I do not mean that psychoanalysts do not take other forms of communication into account, but the terms used to define them tend to be vaguely derogatory: acting, acting out, projection, projective identification are all terms which are regularly accompanied not by an odour of sanctity, but rather by one of disapproval. By the way, why do we say 'odour of sanctity'? Is this not precisely one of those cases in which the original communication, even if transformed later into a verbalisation, was not at an auditory level, but rather at an olfactory one? None of us really thinks that all valid human communication is verbal or verbalisable; the visual arts, music etc. cannot be reduced to words. But the tendency of analysts to assume that all mental activity of any value is potentially verbalisable, and especially that communication occurs at a verbal level, has made more difficult the study of all those phenomena which not only draw strength from underlying non-verbal layers but which sojourn rightfully in those regions. One of the great merits of Neri's book is that it digs up from the underworld a series of illustrations of the richness of human interaction, not taking the word into account, preceding the word and following it.

These self-same characteristics of the contents of *Group* mean that the book can very profitably be read not exclusively by *categories* of people (group and individual psychotherapists, sociologists, philosophers of communication) but by 'individuals', anyone, that is, who knows that being part of a series of groups is a structural aspect of their own 'being human', and wants to know more about it.

Parthenope Bion Talamo

Foreword

This is an extremely interesting book which succeeds in combining erudition with great clarity and a respect of tradition with a refreshing search for new perspectives. It is also a very complex book, full of ideas.

For the reader interested in learning about the developments in the field of group-analysis outside the Anglo-Saxon world this book offers a view of significant work carried out in Italy and in France.

There is no doubt that Neri is very much a psychoanalyst who has arrived to group-analysis from his psychoanalytic base. Psychoanalysis is the main point of reference throughout the book and yet, having chosen to tread the psychoanalytic path, Neri is fascinated by the riches he finds along the way.

The book is crammed with concepts, some of which like 'resonance', 'mirroring', 'basic assumptions' and 'group mind' are well-trodden group concepts taken from Foulkes and Bion. Others like 'group illusion' and 'group skin' are borrowed from Anzieu. Others still, like the idea of 'commuting', although original, derive from Pichon-Riviére's thoughts on how the problems of the individual need to take on a group dimension for transformation to occur. 'Commuting' is a term Neri puts forward to describe how in a group the individual and group aspects alternate in a shuttle motion. Another original concept is the one of 'genius loci' linked to the identity of the group and to its emotional substratum. I found this concept appealing and puzzling at the same time and worth exploring.

Neri illustrates the concepts he presents with references to world literature, philosophy, music and films. This linking of various languages from different corners of the world, from the past to the present, gives the book great breadth and depth as well as a very refreshing atmosphere. I liked the way in which he analyses Mrs Ramsey's character in Virginia Woolf's *To the Lighthouse* from a group perspective.

The book has a very useful glossary at the end listing the most important concepts in the field of group-analysis, followed by an essential bibliography. Besides, Neri introduces inserts throughout the book which contain explanations about key concepts. These two additions are extremely useful and would certainly be helpful for the reader who is not too familiar with the subject matter. The rich clinical sections would also be welcomed by the trainee who is struggling with his first group.

Group goes out of its way to be clear and yet it is also a very academic book. In giving an overall view of the work on groups carried out in Italy and in France, it links Freud, Bion and Foulkes within a group perspective.

Malcolm Pines

Introduction

Psychoanalysis is a discipline which draws attention to questions relating to the quality of our first relationships, to the reasons for anxiety, to what is expressed by symptoms, and memory. How can we help a person to remember what otherwise would be dispersed, or remain fragmentary and marginal? What needs of a child must be satisfied if he is to feel that he exists? What desire urges him towards others? Psychoanalysis has developed particularly refined and delicate instruments to deal with this and other questions. In the course of an analysis, these questions are gathered and linked to each other, they are transformed and adequately located.

If psychoanalysis is seen in this way, the distance separating it from group analysis is not very great. Both in the traditional setting and in that of the group, suffering and illness are considered in the context of a more comprehensive transformation of the personality. In both situations, the therapist leaves space for what is emerging rather than for what has already been formulated, that is to say, he privileges phantasies, dreams, emotions and affects, while refraining from steering the course of events in a predetermined direction. The matter becomes more complex if we wish to refer to particular psychoanalytical theory hypotheses. If the analyst, for example, considers the group as a repetition of the family model composed of father, mother and siblings, and if he intends, within this operative context, to apply the concepts, proper to psychoanalysis, of identification, repression, resistance, reactive formation and fixation, he will certainly be in a position to identify the presence of all these mechanisms in group dynamics, but he will miss the opportunity for picking up the original and specific aspects of the situation. On the contrary, if he goes straight into consideration of the group, and uses models worked through from the starting point of this experience, he will have the chance to make a series of completely new observations which will also throw light on the mechanisms operating in the individual situation.

The choice of method which I have indicated is verified in precise and relevant clinical observations. For example, collective phenomena are active in the group which lead to negative results if the analyst operates in this setting while adopting the same technique used in the dual setting. An example is provided by what happens when using interpretations directed towards individual participants, which in fact activate a collective phenomenology which in the long run dominates and paralyses both the analyst and the members of the group. More precisely, having aroused the basic assumption of dependence, the analyst's words are not taken to be explanations or interpretations, but the utterances of an oracle establishing future destiny, giving rewards and assigning expiations.

The very idea of 'treatment', in the dual situation and in that of the group, refers to partly different schemas. In traditional psychoanalysis, the idea of 'treating' and 'being treated' is linked to an exclusive relationship between therapist and patient. In group analysis, the analysand does not enter into a relationship with the analyst alone, but also with other people, who have an essential role. In fact, anyone who participates in a group takes in the words he hears from the other group members, who he considers his equals, in a different way to those he hears from a figure placed in an asymmetrical position, such as the analyst.

Something similar happens regarding the egocentricity of children, described by Piaget. A child is in a better position to overcome his own egocentricity in the presence of his peers than in the presence of an adult. In fact, when he overcomes his egocentricity with the help of an adult, it often happens that he will fully assume the point of view of the other, but then return to his own. A third observation concerns the differences which exist between the two settings with regard to communication. In the couple and in the group the way in which exchanges take place is different because the dialogue between analyst and analysand is replaced by a circular conversation among a number of people. Moreover, in groups speech necessarily has to cross a 'common space'. A colleague, who was accustomed to working in the traditional (dual) setting, summed up his impressions of his first experience in an analytic group by remarking: 'I was accustomed to playing tennis, and I found myself in a basket-ball team.'

My approach to group analysis is based on some guiding ideas which on the whole provide a theoretical model closely bound up with the clinical aspect.

- The idea that the group constitutes a whole, a community or a collective, capable of thought and emotional working through. When people who take part in a group speak, they naturally do it from a personal point of view. They have begun group analysis because of a need to face up to their problems. However, this is only one aspect of their participation. People who take part in group analysis become a group. As a group, as a 'collective', they carry out the task alongside the analyst, assuming an active role and a joint responsibility for all that concerns living, experiencing and thinking about everything that happens in the common field.

- The idea that group thought operates on elements belonging to a common 'space' or 'field'. In its turn, the field is created and supported by the attention, interest and affective cathexis of the members of the group. The idea of field – as we shall see further on – may be considered from different vertices. For the moment I just want to point out that it is a 'place' in which still unspecified phantasies take shape, a 'special space or relational and mental container' in which emotional transformations and thought operations are carried out.

- The idea that the analyst working in a group has a task which is, in part, different from that which he would assume in the traditional (dual) setting. To the function of interpreter he has to add, with great relevance, that of co-thinker ('leader of the work-group') who expresses himself, as well as in other ways, in creating, maintaining and promoting communication in the group. Conceiving analytic work in the group – which I have indicated with the triad 'group-subject', 'field', 'co-thinker' – finds its natural development and completion in a fourth guiding idea.

- The consideration that the analyst and the members of the group must learn to think in terms of difficulties which emerge in the group field and not in that of single participants.

The small analytic group is made up of a limited number of participants, and each member can form a personal idea of every other member. The participants are facing each other and can at a glance take in, simultaneously, the whole group and each of the participants. The members of the group meet regularly for about two hours, once or preferably twice a week. The therapist is always present at the sessions. The termination of the analysis is not fixed in advance, but a group analysis usually lasts some years. It is preferable that the formation of the group be heterogeneous with regard to symptoms, social and professional position and sphere of interests while a certain homogeneity is useful with regard to age. Some therapists prefer to have a limited number of individual talks with the patients before beginning the group. On the contrary, others entrust the selection of patients to a colleague, or meet the patients directly in the group situation. For my part, I prefer to have talks with each of the possible participants so as to evaluate the group's chances of becoming a therapeutic instrument for individual patients. This choice also gives them the opportunity of getting to know me before they begin to take part in the group.

The design of the book is only partially linear in that it provides for successive stages of investigation which will imply the resumption of themes which have already been treated, in order to consider them from a new perspective which allows more depth and precision.

- The 'Historical Notes' and the first chapter, 'An Overview' are intended to serve as a framework.

- The second part, 'The Group Process', deals with the 'development, history and process of the group' and shows how the group is born and how some of its functions develop. In this part of the book, I examine in particular two moments in the vicissitudes of the group: (1) 'The

Emerging Group State' which corresponds to the first converging of experiences of individual members towards a sensorial area and towards common phantasies; (2) 'The Fraternal Community Stage' which coincides with awareness of being a group and of being able to develop a collective work of knowing and working through.

- The third part, under the general title of 'The Field', continues from the previous section the treatment of the notion of 'The group's Common Space' and places alongside it the concepts of 'The Field' and 'Semiosphere'. This is really a question of three different ways of illustrating the same phenomenon, that of the creation of an area of exchange and working through, common to the members of the group. The Eskimos have 21 different terms for indicating snow, which is of extreme and central importance in their lives, distinguishing between compacted snow, frozen snow, powdery snow and so forth. Similarly, I shall use three terms to illustrate different aspects of what the members of a group share.

- The fourth part of the book is devoted to 'Group Thought'. Some new concepts are proposed, such as the group mind, mimesis and oscillation between thought and affects.

- The fifth part 'Group and Individual', concerns the 'relationship between individuals and the group', and deals in particular with the depersonalisation phenomena which I began to describe when illustrating the 'Emerging Group State'. In the last chapters of this part of the book I also tackle the problem of the relationship between the individual and the field, developing the concepts of 'Commuting' and 'Trans-individual diffusion'.

- The Glossary with the definition of the principal terms used and an Analytic Index complete the book and are intended to facilitate its use as a reference book.

Historical Notes

The use of the group in the 'therapy' of various somatic and psychic illnesses dates back to ancient times and existed before the birth of modern theories on group dynamics. This treatment very often consisted of combined medical and psychological measures within a religious context. For example, in the Asklepeion of Pergamum, in the second century AD, dietetic, thermal and pharmacological treatments were carried out, and group interpretation of dreams by the priests of Aesculapius had a fundamental influence on their choice of prescriptions. The rhetorician Aelius Aristides has left us detailed accounts of this type of treatment in his *Sacred Discourses*.

Group psychoanalysis recognises its descent – through a long series of subsequent experiences and thought – from those first attempts to use the group for therapeutic purposes. However, psychoanalysis seeks not only to provide treatment, but also to develop knowledge about the mental functioning of individuals and groups. Above all, unlike the religious practices mentioned above, psychoanalysis does not aim to obtain miraculous 'cures' by subjecting individuals to a high priest and to the beliefs and superstitions of a group, but attempts to promote a process of healing which involves greater awareness and autonomy.

An interval of fifty years

Keeping the subject within these limits, I should like to point out that the most important ideas for a psychoanalytical approach to the group were worked out over a period of about 50 years, that is to say, the time which elapsed between Freud's *Totem and Taboo* (1912–13) and Bion's *Experiences in Groups* (1961).

During this time there were many changes in the way of considering the group; in fact, there are numerous and significant differences between the group of which Freud speaks and the one in which Bion was interested. The first change has to do with numbers. Freud and other scholars (Le Bon, Trotter, McDougall) who dealt with the subject at the beginning of the century, referred to the mass. On the contrary, Bion (and also Foulkes) turned his attention almost exclusively to small groups, or sub-groups of an organised group (hospital departments, military divisions, etc.). Together with numerical data, motivations changed. For Freud, the study of the masses constituted a part of the effort required to give a unitary base to psychoanalytic psychology. In fact, this was intended to include both individual and collective psychology. On the other hand, Bion and Foulkes, first and foremost, pursued practical ends (rehabilitation, experiments with new therapeutic methods, etc.) and the models which little by little they adopted were more limited and more closely bound up with experience. The main question to which Freud sought an answer was: 'What ties the group together?' This question was the starting point for formulating the theory of libidinal ties and ties of identification in the group. Foulkes and Bion considered the group as a whole, and consequently the question of the tie which keeps the group together lost its importance (see Riccio 1987). Another very relevant question for Freud was whether the Oedipus complex could be considered a basic factor of both the individual psyche and the structure of the group. He thought it could. On the other hand, Bion (1961, p.198) turned his attention to the more primitive levels of mental life, and came to the conclusion that group phenomena cannot be understood by taking the Oedipus complex and family ties as models.

Transference in the group

Passing from a panoramic view to a more specific study, I shall take into consideration a few concepts and authors. It is not my intention to treat the subject exhaustively, but simply to give a few co-ordinates as a framework to this book.

French psychoanalysts have been particularly attentive to the possibility of developing an approach to the group consistent with Freud's formulations and, more generally, with work in the traditional (dual) setting. In this respect, contributions by D. Anzieu and R. Kaës are particularly relevant. Later we shall look at Anzieu's ideas of 'group illusion' and 'the group as a container' and Kaës' concept of 'group associative chain'. For the moment, I would like to mention the use of the transference notion in the group. There is a reason why I want to treat this problem straight away. The use of the transference notion in the group is actually for me a negative point of reference (and I do not base my therapeutic practice on it) rather than a positive one (but I do use it as a starting-point). Since transference is a milestone in psychoanalysis, I want to clear up this question at once.

J. Bejarano (1972, p.17) has dealt in particular with transference in the group, and he specifies four transference objects:

- The monitor or psychotherapist (central transference) who functions as a father-image: at archaic levels (as the infantile Super-ego or cruel father of the horde) or at the Oedipal level (as Super-ego or Ego-ideal).

- The group which functions as a mother-image (Oedipal level) but even more as an archaic mother (archaic level: the horde).

- The others (lateral transference) as a fraternal image.

- The external world, as a place for the projection of individual destructiveness (Thanatos) – but also of Eros (hope of a better world).

Bejarano's aim is to provide the therapist with instruments to help him recognise the affective state of the group and the phantasies which are present from moment to moment. For example, if manifestations of uneasiness and protest occur, the therapist must be in a position to decide whether these manifestations originate from a quest for closeness and affective warmth (Bejarano would speak of transference of a mother-image) or a claim for more freedom of thought (in this case Bejarano would speak of the Oedipal or paternal transference).

Bejarano, in my opinion, raises a relevant question. However, I do not share his idea of using the term and the transference concept to deal with this question. The extrapolation of theoretical constructions from the world of traditional (dual) psychoanalysis to the group – as I pointed out in the introduction – is always problematic. In this case in particular, it can cause confusion and distract attention in an unfortunate way. Transference phenomena, are central to the analytic couple-situation, whereas other phenomena, those relative to the field, are specific to the group. There is also a second reason. It is certainly true that – even in the group setting – there is an affective and phantasmatic cathexis in the therapist, and that various aspects of this cathexis could be likened to transference. This, however, happens within the framework of the group situation and, in my opinion, must be dealt with as one of the elements of this situation. I might add in this regard that the interventions of the group leader most capable of effecting a transformation are not those which interpret the nature of interpersonal relationships (such as transference), but those which deal with the field forces present at that moment. I shall take up this theme in greater detail in the Appendix to my book (p.147) when I deal with the therapeutic potentiality of group analysis.

Foulkes

Bion and Foulkes work at passing from a viewpoint which sees the group as a certain number of people in association (a plurality held together by a leader or by an ideal) to one that places emphasis on its unity. Bion developed this idea on the basis of K. Lewin's thought and on *Gestaltpsycologie* ('the whole is different from the sum of the parts'), Foulkes mainly on the basis of studies concerning nerve networks. On this subject Foulkes writes (1964, p.70; 1948, p.140):

> This concept [of group unity], which is characteristic of the group-analysis approach, seems difficult to grasp and people seem reluctant to use it operationally. What we have in mind is not just the sum of relationships between individuals interacting in a group, but more of a real psychological entity.

> The group as a whole is not simply a turn of phrase, it is a living organism, as distinct from the individuals comprising it. It has moods and reactions, a spirit, a feeling and an atmosphere.

In this context we can speak of a matrix, of a communication network. This network is not merely interpersonal but could rightly be described as transpersonal and supra-personal.

Foulkes considers the group being as a network. Every knot can be imagined as a person, linked by a strand (a relationship) to the other persons and to the net as a whole. The network, in fact, is not simply a sum of two way relationships, but has the characteristics of a whole which are different from those of the strands. (see Bria 1986).

Network

The idea of a net can lead us to various types of reference – social, biological, family, etc. 'The individual is a part of a social network, a small nodal part, so to speak, of this network, and can only be considered in isolation in an artificial way, like a fish out of water. Besides these horizontal ramifications, with other people and with the community, the individual has a vertical connection which represents his biological heritage, which he develops throughout his whole life.'

Thinking in terms of network also leads us to consider the question of illness from a new point of view. 'Somatic and psychic illnesses are not simply a function of the individual's personality, even as symptoms, but are a function of an entire plexus of an entire network of relationships between many individuals.'

Even in a small analytic group there is a network involving the participant and the therapist (see Foulkes 1948, p.42; Foulkes and Anthony 1957, p.54 and p.258).

Underlying the network is the matrix of the group from which the network evolves. Foulkes (1964, p.292) suggests a general definition: 'The matrix is the common shared ground which ultimately determines the meaning and significance of all events and upon which all communications and interpretations, verbal and non-verbal, rest. This concept links up with that of communication.'

G. Lo Verso and M. Papa (1992) elaborate Foulkes' concept of the matrix from three accepted meanings:

1. *The basic matrix:* represents the presupposition of communication, the unifying substrate whose presence allows the immediate possibility of understanding.

2. *The dynamic matrix:* forms within the group situation as a specific aspect of that group and not another, and is, except in the case of 'rigidity', in perennial transformation.

3. *The personal matrix*: concerns the individual, and is formed on the basis of his experience of forming part of a group, the original family one, of which he has incorporated an entire set of relationships, not to mention the significance, myth-making and phantasy-weaving aspects of these relationships.

To illustrate the sense of the idea of matrix, alongside these definitions by Foulkes and Lo Verso and Papa, we may access the evocative capacity of the word itself. Speaking of 'matrix' (and not mother) means likening the group to the image of an ovary (in which there are numerous egg-cells) and to that of germinative soil. The generative dimension of the group, the fact that it contains elements which are not yet individuated but can take shape, becomes evident. The word 'matrix' also has cultural overtones. For example, one may wonder about one's own matrix, or ask someone else, 'What is your matrix?' The question does not require an answer indicating precise notions or explanations about specific formation, but rather that the person should speak about his ideas, feelings, attitudes and values, which are the basis of the group or society in which he has grown up (see Menarini and Pontalti 1984).

Bion

Foulkes speaks of network and matrix, Bion of the mental states (mentality) of the group.

Just as there are regressive and evolutive aspects of the personality in the individual, there is in the group a regressive mentality (which in some measure corresponds to Freud's mass-group) and an evolutive mentality (shown, for example, in a capacity to co-operate in order to attain an end).

To develop the notion of work-group (or rational group), Bion takes his inspiration from McDougall's idea of the organised group. McDougall maintains that if certain conditions are fulfilled, those united in a group can develop a capacity for thought comparable to that of an isolated individual.

The organised group

W. McDougall (1927) writes: 'Participation in the life of a group degrades the individual, making his mental processes similar to those of the crowd, whose brutality, inconsistency and unreasoning impulsiveness have been the themes of many many writers. Nevertheless it is only by participating in group life that man can become completely human, that he can raise himself above the level of a savage.' (p.20)
(continued)

The organised group (continued)

The solution of this paradox rests on the organisation of the group. Organisation controls degrading tendencies and, in the best cases, gives a helping hand to group life thanks to which man can rise a little above the animals.

According to McDougall, the conditions which allow a group to become an organised group are as follows. The first, on which all the rest are based, is a certain degree of continuity in the existence of the group. The second condition is that an adequate idea of the nature, composition, functions and capacity of the group, should be formed in the mind of the mass of members of the group. A third condition, perhaps not absolutely essential, is the interaction (especially in the form of conflict and rivalry) of the group with other similar groups, animated by different ideals and aims, and dominated by different traditions and customs. In the fourth place it is necessary that a body of traditions, customs and habits, determining the relations of the members to each other and to the group as a whole, should exist in the members' minds (see Cruciani 1983, pp.21–36).

Unlike McDougall, Bion considers the 'work-group' not as something which is created if the opportune conditions are achieved, but as an ever-present mental dimension, even if it has to be developed and reinforced through discipline and effort. In fact, according to Bion, both the mentality of the work-group and primitive mentality correspond to man's ethological endowments as a social animal. The fact that the members of the group are united is not the cause of the work-group mentality (as it is not the cause of primitive mentality) but only a condition which brings it to light.

There is a second important difference between McDougall and Bion. The emphasis which McDougall places on organisation sets his theory in the sociological rather than the psychological. The organised group is, above all, a form of social relationship. On the other hand, Bion places himself completely within the dimension of psychology. The work-group is a collective mentality and at the same time an aspect of the individual mind.

The terms 'rational group' and 'work-group' correspond to two chronological moments and two stages of Bion's development. To begin with he speaks of a 'group with a rational structure', referring to those aspects of collective mental life which maintain a level of behaviour linked with reality, such as the awareness of the passing of time and the ability to follow methods which may be roughly called scientific. Such methods may still be rudimentary (like that of the monkey using a stick to reach a banana) but they are different from simple motor activity (like that of a monkey flinging itself against the bars) and from the automatism of actions promoted by primitive mentality.

Bion later (1961, p.106) replaced the name 'rational group' with 'work-group'. As he himself says: 'In some groups with which I was concerned, what I had called "rational group" was spontaneously called "work-group". The name is concise, and since it expresses well an aspect of the phenomenon which I wish to describe, from now on I shall use this term.' The phrase 'work-group' used by Bion makes it clear that a learning activity is necessary if a participant is to be able to make a contribution to the achievement of the group's aims. This term also shows that participation in the work-group implies having developed some skills which Freud had indicated as characteristic of the individual's Ego, that is, attention, verbal representation and symbolic thought.

The second group mentality described by Bion is primitive mentality. Primitive mentality corresponds to the tendency to give automatic replies. It is a dimension in which it is hard not to become completely involved. To illustrate this characteristic I shall tell the tale of a friend with a sense of humour:

> My first contact with politics was one day many years ago in a time of unrest. I was at Middle School. I was very proud to have had this first encounter with politics, and anxious to tell my family all about it.
>
> When I went home to lunch, I met my brothers and my father, an elderly gentleman of liberal education. Full of enthusiasm, I began to tell them that the Grammar School boys had arrived, and that we had gone in a procession to the other schools to get the boys to come out. We had gone all round the town. My father asked me: 'What were the reasons for the demonstration? What did you want?'
>
> I replied: 'I don't know, but we were all shouting "Fast-Bell, Fast-Bell".'
>
> My brothers burst out laughing. It took me some time to understand that I had joined the procession out of step. In fact they were shouting: 'Bel-fast, Bel-fast!'

The more the group functions according to primitive mentality, the more limited is the space for the individual. It is important for the therapist to be aware of this, and in particular of the fact that the group can limit people's liberty by requiring them to adjust to a certain collective functioning. This adjustment is demanded both regarding thought (through the elimination of dissonant thoughts) and emotion. For instance, the group may exert coercion in the sense that everyone must be happy and show themselves to be so. If those forces which tend to limit freedom to express oneself and to think prevail, then individuals lose their uniqueness and become interchangeable. Therefore, the group therapist's task is not to oblige individuals to form a group (as in the case of a mass group) but to slow down processes that are too swift and disruptive, and to underline the peculiarities, differences and rights of the individuals.

According to Bion, primitive mentality is supported and pervaded by three phantasies which alternate in the group. Bion defines them as 'basic assumptions' to indicate how fundamental and indisputable they are. In a 1991 paper his daughter Parthenope Bion Talamo speaks about them as follows:

In a broad outline of Bion's theory, he declares that the attempts made by human beings united in a group to develop creative conduct (in whatever field) may be disturbed and even completely broken off by the emergence of thoughts and emotions rooted in unconscious phantasies concerning the 'true' motives for the foundation of the group.

There are three main classes into which these phantasies fall. 1) 'religious', the phantasy of depending totally on an absolute and dominant figure. 2) that of 'coupling' according to which the group is said to be formed with the sole aim of reproduction, a class which merges into the religious one when the product of the mating, whether it be a person or an idea, is seen as a Messiah who is still to come. 3) Fight/flight, a basic phantasy according to which the group gets together in order to deal exclusively with its own preservation, and this depends exclusively on attacking the enemy in mass or in fleeing from it. (1991)

In Bion's (1961) description in *Experiences in Groups* the two mentalities (work-group mentality and primitive mentality) are presented as co-present and opposing. In other words, primitive mentality and the work-group mentality do not constitute a sequence. The evolved man (expression of the work-group) and the regressed man (expression of primitive mentality) are present in both the caveman and his modern descendant, technological man. Actually, in technological man, the primitive mentality – if it does not meet adequate opposition in the work-group – is all the more dangerous in so far as it is masked by a sophisticated logic and endowed with immeasurable power.

The active presence of the work-group mentality and primitive mentality, both in the group and in each of the participants, puts the individual in a situation of insoluble conflict. If he participates in the work-group, he feels deprived of warmth and strength, if he adheres to the group as a basic assumption, he knows he may find it impossible to pursue his own ends as a thinking and reflecting individual. Participating in a group dominated by primitive mentality is revitalising, even when it leads to catastrophe, while when we detach ourselves from our herding nature, we suffer a sense of limitation, we realise how deeply dependent on others we are and we feel alone.

On the other hand, this conflict between work-group and primitive mentality is also essential, and it is the origin of transformations. In Bion's opinion there is no true growth where the evolutional aspect is detached from the primitive aspect. It is only when what is evolved comes into resonance with what is primitive, and drags it out of its isolation that there is real development of the group and of the personality of the individual. I shall take up these themes again in Chapter 8, which is devoted to the difference between brain and mind, and in Chapter 12, relating to transformations in 'K' (knowledge) and transformations in 'O' (evolution of what is 'primitive').

relating to transformations in 'K' (knowledge) and transformations in 'O' (evolution of what is 'primitive').

Observations

In considering the group I have been deeply influenced by the idea of the group as a totality (unity of the group) and in particular by Bion's view of collective mental states (mentality). In my opinion, these ideas are not in conflict with the attention which the therapist must pay to individuals, to their vicissitudes and their experiences.

Another great influence has been the concept of the matrix, which has numerous points of contact with the development of the group's common space and of the field. More specifically, the idea contained in Foulkes' concept of the matrix seems to me to be useful. That is to say, to look for the constituent elements of the common space and of the group field in sensorial experiences, and consider that the group's life is planted in a germinative terrain (field taken as a morphogenetic field). As far as the opposition between primitive mentality and work-group are concerned, I am convinced that Bion's description of primitive mentality and the strong bi-partition which he establishes between basic assumptions and the work-group is valuable in group analytic work as a compass to steer by in moments of crisis and confusion. At such times the analyst has to resist all temptation to conform to the 'tensions' and the feelings which are dominating the group, and assume the responsibility of thinking as an individual. Nevertheless, if these notions are constantly assumed as the axes on which the therapist bases his interventions, they may give the idea of an analyst who is too ideal, severe and intransigent. The group therapist is also a co-thinker working side by side with the other participants, and not someone who is in some way detached or on another level.

I should add that even though Bion's idea regarding the existence of a work-group mentality may have had less success than that of primitive mentality (basic assumptions), I maintain that the two notions are inseparable. I also think that the group therapist should devote to the development of the work-group at least as much, if not more, attention, as he does to the analysis of those phenomena which are proper to primitive mentality. In fact, group thought is both a product and an expression of the work-group.

PART 1

Analytic Work

CHAPTER I

An Overview

In this chapter which I still consider to be an introduction, I shall examine four 'objects of the analyst's attention', giving the same consideration and space to each. My aim is to provide a panorama of the complex work that goes on during the sessions of group analysis.

In subsequent chapters I shall deal mostly with the last two objects (the relationship between individuals and the group, and trans-personal phenomena) because they have been studied least, and the other two objects of the analyst's attention (individuals and interpersonal relationships) will remain somewhat in the background.

During the session, as I have said, the analyst must keep in mind four elements, moving his attention from one to the other so as to create adequate links between them. These elements are:

- individuals
- interpersonal relationships
- relationships between individuals and the group
- trans-personal phenomena.

Before dealing with the subject of this chapter, I should like to point out once more that the relationship between individuals and the group will be taken up again in Chapters 9, 10 and 11, when I shall deal with group thought. The treatment of trans-personal phenomena will be developed within the notion of the field in Chapter 6, after I have introduced the concept of the group's common space in Chapter 4.

Individuals

During the course of therapy, each participant puts forward his own phantasy history, using different forms of expression, such as stories, dreams, behaviour, etc. Each of his interventions is linked to the on-going activity of the group, but it is also linked up to his previous interventions, following the main drift of his phantasies.

The psychoanalyst recognises the principal features of each intervention. He notices how each of the persons evolves at the same pace as the relationship he has established with him and with the group. He makes a mental note of how individual patients use the responses they obtain during therapy and of whether there is a development (or a block) in the evolution of their personality.

Listening to the persons in a group in an analytic way is similar to listening to certain pieces of music, such as *Peter and the Wolf.* Prokofiev's work is composed in such a way that the listener can hear not only the timbre and the sound of a certain instrument, but also how there are certain musical phrases which correspond to it and identify it in the orchestra, and how the instrument gradually develops these. In a similar way, it is important for the therapist to recognise the abilities of individuals and their particular styles. This recognition also functions as an antidote to transformation of the group into a mass. Tocqueville reminds us that: 'A group cannot be free if its members are not free.'

I should like to add that the psychoanalyst does not direct his attention only to those members of the group who are actually speaking. For a positive development of the therapy, it is equally important, or perhaps even more so, that he also turns his attention to those who are not able to express themselves in words. By linking together in his mind short phrases, facial expressions and fragments of feeling and thought, he can help to form an 'ability to be subjects' which these patients, who may be confused or contradictorily plural – do not possess or only potentially possess (see Cuomo 1986). To illustrate the contribution which the analyst can make in helping those patients who cannot express themselves to become subjects, I might imagine the relationship between a father and a son who is undecided which faculty to enter because it is difficult for him to determine what he might become in adult life. The father thinks: 'My son ought to become an engineer.' This thought will probably move the son to reject precisely this profession. However, the interest shown by the father – who has shouldered the problem of a comprehensive and forward-looking image for his son – provides him with a point of reference and orientation. This point of reference may be negative (i.e. rejected by the son) but it nevertheless helps the latter to form ideas.

Interpersonal relationships

If this were the only dimension of analytic work in groups, analysis in the traditional setting and analysis in the group setting would be similar. In fact, the only difference would be that there would not be just two people in the room (an analyst and an analysand) but 7, 8 or even 15 people (one being the analyst). Group analysis would therefore give the impression of being 'analysis in parallel' (or 'analysis in a group') of different analysands, and the group would be the frame within which the analysis takes place. This is the approach proposed by Schilder (in the USA) and Wolf and Schwartz (in Great Britain) who work with this very technique, commonly called 'analysis in a group'.

Analysis in a group

Working with this approach places the emphasis on individual transference relationships. The patients receive the interpretations and responses which they would receive if they were in the traditional (couple) setting. The psychotherapist directs the therapeutic work towards transference and resistances in a very active way.

The sessions are frequent, usually four times a week. Two of these are alternate sessions – that is to say sessions without the therapist. The emergence of a group process does not receive the analyst's attention which is focused to a large extent on the individual participants. In any case the therapist makes very limited use of group dynamics (see Brown and Pedder 1991, p.121; Wolf and Schwartz 1972, pp.41–91).

However, the group is not only a frame. During sessions there are usually very free and lively exchanges about what is happening and what each member of the group is communicating, both consciously and unconsciously.

The other members of the group are frequently able to grasp aspects of the experience of the person who is speaking which he himself either does not recognise or does so only partially. Their perceptions are both precise and selectively distorted. They are precise perceptions because, as I mentioned, the members of the group almost always succeed in grasping the active phantasy nucleus. They are distorted, because they are supported by strong identifications and intense affective cathexis. The background atmosphere of the group also plays an important role. If tolerance and friendliness predominate in the group, correctness of perception prevails over any distortion. If on the contrary there is a persecutory atmosphere in the group, then perception becomes greatly distorted.

To illustrate the capacity of the participants in a group to grasp the emotions and experiences of the other members, Foulkes (1948) used a term taken from physics: 'resonance'.

Resonance

Acoustic resonance was discovered in about 1450. In 1862 Helmholtz gener-alised the concept after observing that the same phenomenon was produced in optics, in electromagnetism etc., that is to say, wherever there were vibrations. A physical system can be set vibrating even on a frequency very distant from its own, or from its natural frequencies. The effect remains weak but increases as the excitant frequency approaches the natural one and reaches a very large am-plitude of vibration (amplitude of resonance) when it reaches one of the natural frequencies (resonance frequency): the system is then said to be 'in resonance'.

In the group, too, there may be a generic emotional contact, which corre-sponds to what in physics is resonance at a long distance from natural frequen-cies. However, true resonance between two or more persons (system in resonance) is produced on a particular theme, phantasy or sentiment (see An-zieu 1976, pp.340–341).

Resonance between members of the group is the foundation of group work. The leader of the group must encourage it, for example by pointing out similarities in ways of expressing oneself or by clarifying any misunderstandings. I.D. Yalom (1970, p.116) writes about this function of the analyst:

> A member of a group of mine, a jazz pianist, once made observations about the role of the therapist, saying that at one time, at the beginning of his career, he had tremendously admired the virtuosi of some instrument or other. It was only much later that he matured enough to realise that really great jazz musicians are those who know how to bring out the sounds made by others, who know how to keep quiet and how to make the whole complex work.

It is also true that resonance between two or more participants in a group always requires a certain emotive working through. A member of the group may, for example, have a dream for another participant. Just as a mother-bird pre-digests food for her young, he assumes as his own the emotional situation which another member of the group is not in a position to work through for himself, and repre-sents it in dream-images which he then brings into the session. Kaës (1985, pp.91–100) expresses a very similar idea when he writes: 'Transformations which certain members of the group are not able to complete are developed (by the ana-lyst or by another member of the group) just as a mother detoxicates her child's internal space thanks to her function of holding and transforming.'

Moreover there is always a self-knowledge value in entering into resonance with and metabolising another participant's states of mind. Sometimes this func-tion of self-knowledge is pre-eminent. In this case we can speak of a 'mirror-effect'. A mirror-effect appears in a characteristic way 'when a certain

number of individuals meet and react to each other. An individual sees himself –
often the repressed part of himself – reflected in the interaction of the other members of the group. He sees them react in the same way as he reacts himself, or in
contrast with his behaviour. In this way he learns to know himself through the
effect he has on the others and through the image which they have formed of him'
(see Foulkes 1964, p.121).

It is not only between two people that resonance and the mirror-effect develop.
Sometimes associative and working-through chains are created to which most of
the group members contribute. In this case, the activity of metabolising and working through is like the unravelling of a dialogue with several voices.

The associative chain in the group

Free association is an integral part of psychoanalytic technique used to penetrate to the unconscious levels of the mind. For obvious reasons, this technique
cannot be used extensively in the group setting. However, on certain occasions
the group in its characteristic free-flowing discussions can get near to it. These
discussions can lead, and fairly frequently do in well-functioning analytic
groups, to the unexpected emergence of a chain activity, to which each member
contributes an essential and specifically personal link. This event may deepen
the level of communication and lead to developments in the dynamics of the
group.

The group associative chain is a way of expressing phantasies of individual
participants and of the group as a whole, which otherwise would be difficult to
express.

These chains are brought about in two ways. They are formed from successive or similar statements by members of the group, and they are determined by
a group logic, where contents and structurising methods reveal group thought
(see Foulkes and Anthony 1957, p.151; Kaës 1993).

Interaction between individuals and the group

Just as the image of the associative chain throws light on one aspect of group communication, another image may account for a second feature of such
communication and this is the star-shaped image of the group. All the members
are linked together, not along a chain, but to a central point which acts as a con-
nector and a centre.

This centre may already be known and set up. For example, it may be a phantasy, an emotion, the central feeling of the session, with which everyone
establishes a connection. However, it may also be as yet unknown and waiting to
be defined. I am reminded of an Islamic story of the Sufi tradition.

There was once a country where no one had ever seen an elephant. The King of India, who for political reasons wanted to make an alliance with the king of that country, sent him as a gift an elephant, which arrived at night and was immediately enclosed in a pavilion in the embassy garden. The people's curiosity was great, and in order to see what an elephant looked like, four of the bravest men decided to creep secretly into the pavilion while it was dark. So as not to be found out, they did not take a lantern with them, but simply touched the animal, feeling it carefully and then quickly running back to their friends who were impatiently waiting for them.

'This is what an elephant is like,' said the first, who had touched a foot, 'it is like a completely round column.'

But the second, who had touched its trunk, retorted, 'Not at all; it is like a thick rope, very thick and very long.'

The third, who had carefully felt one of the elephant's ears, assured them that the animal was like a great fan, and the fourth, who had examined the tail, asserted that at the end of the day the elephant was just like a pig's tail, but much higher up and rougher.

The story of 'The Elephant in the Dark' warns us not to 'speak about things without having a global view of them' (see Mandel 1992). However, as in many Sufi stories, another reading is also possible. We can in fact imagine the four explorers discussing with each other what they had felt and thought when touching the elephant, and their companions who had remained outside the pavilion not just simply listening, but adding their own opinions and hypotheses. The story then becomes an illustration of the star-shaped group, and is like an invitation to take account of the comparison of different vertices in order to gain a knowledge of something which is too hard for a single person to take in. For a single person, in fact, it may be hard to think about so many different points of view, whereas if each is represented by a member of the group, everyone can benefit at the same time from these differing perspectives.

Transpersonal phenomena

The last of the four 'subjects of attention' of the analyst – transpersonal phenomena – is in reality something which is extensive, diffusive, impalpable, and difficult to pinpoint. To make it clearer, I shall distinguish between three orders of transpersonal phenomena which appear to overlap in the clinical situation. They are:

- the atmosphere or 'background tone' of the session
- the medium
- the effects of primitive mentality and basic assumptions.

I shall now speak a little about each of these phenomena.

- *Atmosphere*: the participants in a group share a combination of experiences, emotions and bodily sensations which they themselves originate. By a combining effect (synaesthesia) these elements tend to appear as a diffusive and mobile 'whole' which is perceived as the atmosphere of the group. Fritz Redl defines it as 'the tonality of the basic feeling which underlies the life of a group, the sum of the emotions of each individual, in confrontation with the others, towards work and towards the institution, towards the group as a unit and towards the external world'.

- *Medium*: McLuhan (1977, pp.25–30) states that the media through which communication occurs are never neutral towards this same communication, but on the contrary influence it deeply. Sometimes the impact of the medium even dominates that of the content which it should be conveying: 'the medium is the message'. The introduction of a new medium or a change in the medium modifies the perception of those who are experiencing it. For example, the fact that in a room the light dims or brightens or that there is more or less noise, represents changes of medium. When such changes are slow, there is a greater possibility of adaptation than when the changes are rapid. In the latter case the result is that the area of perceptive relationship to the medium becomes cloudy and partially anaesthetised. This perceptive area may even be completely excluded from consciousness. The overall effect is a more or less intense feeling of unreality. Pribram gives us an example of phenomena brought about by the impact of a change of medium. It concerns something which happened in New York.

> The police noticed that in a certain area, from a certain date, there had been a considerable increase in night calls. These calls, which were for various reasons (fear of burglary, suspicion of attempts at rape, uneasiness, fear of gas leaks, etc.), were found to be without foundation. From further study of this phenomenon it was possible to discover that the "unfounded calls" were concentrated within three or four periods of the night. This observation led to the explanation of the phenomenon. These times, in fact, coincided with the timetable of a night-time underground train which had been cancelled. The alarm calls corresponded to the deafening silence left by the missing train. (see Bruni and Nebbiosi 1987, pp.79–90)

The situation of the small analytic group is in itself a new medium for those coming to take part in it. I shall deal with this phenomena at greater length and with the depersonalisation experiences deriving from it in the next chapter, which is devoted to the Emerging state of the group. What I want to mention now is that a particularly important element of the medium of small analytic groups is the presence (physical or somatic) of all the members of the group. When one of the members is missing (when there is an empty place), this absence is perceived as a change in the medium. Clinical experience indicates that in such cases, if group communication is to be re-established in a satisfactory way, the change (the absence) which weighs down on the group must be adequately worked through.

- Primitive mentality and basic assumptions: I have already mentioned primitive mentality and basic assumptions in the 'Historical Notes'. I should like at this point simply to emphasise that it is, properly speaking, a question of 'systems', which distort the perception of events.

Technique

It is difficult to recognise the atmosphere and the effects of the medium and those of basic assumptions, because these phenomena are camouflaged in the environment of the group.

Therefore it is essential that the analyst should succeed in not being the 'good analyst' which the participants in the group expect him to be, and that he should manage to keep open the option to feel and think things that may appear to the members of the group and even to himself to be useless, 'offensive' and irrelevant.

The analyst may even entrust the picking up and recognising of transpersonal phenomena to the artistic side of his personality. These transpersonal 'effects', in fact, are more easily perceived by a mind capable of being moved and surprised than by the rational mind. To illustrate this point I shall not relate a story, but a personal memory, which is particularly evocative.

> I remember a Polish lady who lived in exile in Rome. At a certain time of the year, this lady used to cry. I realised later that her crying was to do with the flowering of the lime-trees. There was an abundance of these trees in the Polish town she came from. I had never been aware of the presence of the scent of lime-trees in Rome, because in my city these trees are rare and not very popular. However, from that time on I have come to recognise the sweet and pervasive scent of lime-trees in the complex and confused environment of Rome.

PART 2

The Group Process

In the last chapter I spoke of the four 'objects of the analyst's attention'. To clarify the picture I must add another element. At the centre of the analyst's interests, besides the four 'objects' I mentioned, there is also the history of the group. The group has its own vicissitudes, which are interwoven with the vicissitudes of the persons who take part in it, but do not identify with them. Whereas, on the contrary, the vicissitudes of the individuals occur within the framework of the group's history.

In particular, there are two crucial moments over which I shall linger because they are very important in determining the analytic functioning of a small group. These 'crucial moments' are:

- the Emerging group state
- the Fraternal Community stage.

The Emerging group state is particularly significant because in this phase the group starts to become a coherent unit. The Fraternal Community stage is important because it is the moment in which the group is constituted in its full sense as a collective subject capable of thought and working through. This section of the book, besides the two chapters devoted to the Emerging group state and Fraternal Community stage, contains two more chapters, 'The Group's Common Space' and 'Genius Loci' which illustrate particular aspects of the phenomenology of the Emerging group state, regarding the boundary of the group and the contextual creation of the 'group's common space'.

CHAPTER 2

The Emerging Group State

I shall now deal with three components of the complex phenomenology of the Emerging group state, that is, waiting for the Messiah, group illusion and experiences of depersonalisation. I shall deal later with the problems of group boundaries in the chapter regarding the creation of the group's common space.

Waiting for the Messiah and group illusion

Every group is built around the idea of a Messiah, around a fascinating and enthralling idea and around the person who supplies it. In the small analytic group the Messianic idea (psychoanalysis) is tied up with the figure of the analyst. It is precisely because it originates from the receiving and utilising of a particular heritage of ideas, that of psychoanalysis, that the small analytic group nourishes within itself a powerful vein of Messianic hope, of confidence in the future and the possibility of greatly enriching one's view of the world (see Correale 1992).

However, the Emerging group state is characterised by illusion as well as by Messianic hope. In the beginning stages of the group, for example, we often hear assertions like 'we are good, we are the best group in the world', assertions which are not based on a realistic judgement of the functioning of the group, but on a collective illusion. The group analyst is tempted to join in this euphoria, which gratifies him (if the group is a good group, surely this is proof that the analyst is a good analyst!). However, he must resist this temptation. Group illusion is a response to a desire for security, a desire to preserve a threatened ego. The preservation of identity moves from the individual to the group, group illusion responds to the threat to individual narcissism by setting up group narcissism. In this way the group finds its identity and at the same time the narcissistic union of all members within the group's good breast is confirmed. The aim of forming a group and of forming a good group, constitutes a defensive movement away from the real – sought yet feared – object of psychotherapy, which is to bring everyone individually into question (see de Martis and Barale 1993).

What I have just illustrated is one aspect of 'group illusion', and highlighting only this aspect of the problem would give a partial view. In fact, I believe that group illusion must be taken into consideration, not only on account of its negative aspects and its resistance to analytic work, but also because it is a way of responding to the urgent need of members of the group to stay together even if they still lack the ability to form a relationship. While they are still unable to form a group of people who can work together, they may, nevertheless, be together as if they were in a dream, on waking, each going his own way, each speaking his own language, which is incomprehensible to the others.

So, group illusion has several facets. It is a reaction to total anguish and bewilderment, but it is also an initial condition for birth and development (see Anzieu 1976, pp.312–317).

Depersonalisation

Alongside these phenomena, together with colleagues of the Research Centre on groups, 'Il Pollaiolo', I have been able to bring to light the importance and significance of the emergence of phenomena of depersonalisation and deindividualisation in the Emerging state of the group. The view on which we concentrated our attention is different from the one described by Bion when speaking of primitive mentality, because it corresponds to a particular moment of the group's existence (the Emerging state) and not to a stable dimension of the group's life. In particular, we have been able to observe how, to a certain degree, phenomena of the Emerging state of the group are habitually experienced by members of a small group as a loss of the boundaries of Self. This sense of loss is accompanied by experiencing change in their way of thinking and of relating to surrounding reality (see Palmieri 1988).

It is as though their feelings and expectations were no longer localised, but were diffused in a common or shared space.

Similar feelings occur in the passage from sleep to waking: Where is my head? Are my feet in the right place? Was I here when I fell asleep? A condition caused by slight alcoholic drunkenness is similar to the sensation of loss of boundaries in the Emerging group state. It is easy for the mind to produce images, emotions and bodily experiences that the subject feels refer not so much to himself, as to the context in which he is immersed. The experience of change in one's normal way of being and of 'relating to others', is also shown, for example, when noticing how time loses its normal everyday dimension. Space seems to acquire new and previously unknown connotations. Having a particular relationship with objects gives way to a certain indistinction between subject and object. There is no detachment from experience, but neither is there the possibility of directing one's own participation in a voluntary and active way. Many members refer – but only later on – to dreams or phantasies about journeys in countries without time or history, with landscapes that are at once both familiar and unfamiliar.

These mental states, although they do not correspond to any precise phantasy, are nevertheless very captivating. The common experience of the group in the 'Emerging state' is much more powerful than the pre-existing mental state of the individual members. Each member not only syntonises with these common mental states, but is captivated by them. Moreover, each member contributes involuntarily to determining them. We might take as an example the moment when at a party the guests no longer remain isolated, but are caught up in the mounting excitement, they are already at one with the group and the reigning atmosphere, but still retain a certain memory of their previous position.

A crossroads

These phenomena of depersonalisation and loss of reality – such as occur in the group illusion – are not a stable condition, but represent a situation of transit towards other conditions. In some cases they lead to a condition of paralysis where thinking is impossible. Those present are involved in a globalising and confusing situation where the sense of their own identity is diminished or lost entirely. In this case it is correct to speak, in a narrow sense, of depersonalisation and non-fulfilment effect.

It is often a painful experience. For example, in one group the members began to dream repeatedly that 'the whole group had been transformed into a mirror' thus indicating the need to 'get on the outside' and be shown 'what they were like one by one' in order to emerge from a disturbing condition.

On the other hand, in certain cases we need to speak of 'deindividualisation' rather than 'depersonalisation'. The picture here is not one of 'destructurisation', but of 'disassembly' of individual perceptive, communicative and behavioural schemas which gradually slip away without effort or constriction.

This process (of disassembly) is directed at constructing group schemes and activating adequate collective modes of elaboration and thought. Their thought becomes more associative as each participant takes up the words of those who have spoken before him. What they talk about refers to the situation which is being experienced in the group at that moment. It is this very parallel and almost contemporaneous activating of collective modes of functioning which protects the members of the group from an excess of depersonalisation (see Correale and Parisi 1979, p.60).

Technique

One technique, which used to be prescribed for the analyst, particularly at the beginning of group analytic work, and which now appears somewhat dated, was that he should be silent, detached, and postpone his interpretation, all of which did not allow the group to be helped to emerge from the difficulties connected with this phase. I remember the first *T-group* I conducted many years ago.

> With other colleagues I had been invited to organise a training group for teachers in religious schools. In my group I remained impassive. The situation was in a certain sense paradoxical because, facing an impassive group analyst, there were elementary school-masters and nuns from small country towns in Sicily, who were bewildered and undecided.

> During the second session, the sun was beating down on the nape of my neck, yet I continued motionless and saying nothing until a little nun got up and drew the curtain. That was the end of my career as an impassive and detached analyst. The closing of the curtain led me to think that there must have been many feelings in the group, and it would have been better to have found a way to help them circulate.

My present point of view on technique in the phase of the Emerging state of the group is very different. I now realise more fully the difficulties which participation in a group creates for its members. Bion compares the emotional intensity and problematics of the first confrontation with a group to the initial relationship of a newborn baby with the breast. In a small group, for example, members might find it enormously difficult to speak to and understand each other. Whoever ventures to break the silence feels that in speaking he is running a risk, a risk of falling into a void with nothing to hold on to.

In the second place I realise that, like the other participants, I must be well aware that I too am subject to powerful emotions proper to the Emerging state of the group, and that, just like the others, I may feel disorientated and have difficulty in thinking. I too may sometimes be tempted to isolate myself from the more confused aspects of my experience. I am, however, quite determined not to shield myself (and I do not think I could shield myself) from these experiences.

In any case, I cannot submit to them passively. On the contrary, I behave like a diver plunging into the Emerging state of the group and then re-emerging from the depths. Re-emerging and catching my breath, I have to remember pauses for decompression, and even prolong these because I have to wait for my less experienced fellow-divers to follow me to the surface. Bion speaks of what I call 'decompression' in terms of the analyst's *reverie* and α-*function*.

The α-function

The alpha function proposed by Bion corresponds to an unknown variable to which we assign transforming operations acting on all sensorial and emotional experiences, both waking and sleeping.

The absence or inversion of the alpha function not only makes it impossible to distinguish between conscious and unconscious, but also to produce thought. The untransformed sensorial and emotional elements (beta elements) are in fact experienced as objects and ejected into the surrounding field (somatic or environmental).

The structure of the baby's alpha function is closely linked to its relationship with its mother and her capacity for love and understanding. Thanks to her alpha function the mother 'digests' the sensorial impressions which the baby, who is still immature, is unable to metabolise.

With a more direct reference to the analytic situation, we can say that the alpha function is tied up with reverie. This means it is tied up with 'the analyst's capacity to receive the patient's verbal or pre-verbal communications, a receptive capacity which is accompanied by a working-through activity' (see Corrao 1981, pp.29–30; D'Apruzzo 1987; Di Chiara 1992).

CHAPTER 3

The Fraternal Community Stage

In the last chapter I illustrated the phenomena of the Emerging state of the group (waiting for a Messiah, group illusion, depersonalisation) which represent on the one hand the reactions of the members on their first encounter with the group situation, and on the other the beginnings of a shared collective situation.

In this chapter I shall look at a different phase of the group history, which may follow the emerging phase, but perhaps only after months or years of work. This is the phase in which there is a growing awareness of the existence and working potential of the group as a collective subject, and as a community capable of thought (see Resnik 1983).

Jean-Paul Sartre

Jean-Paul Sartre suggests that there is a moment of fusion which transforms what has up to then been 'a certain number of people' into a coherent and superpersonal whole. After this fusion has come about, the people who form the group talk of themselves as 'we'; they are capable of operating as a group, they stop simply being numbers in a series and establish reciprocal relationships.

Awareness of being a group

Sartre declares that the constitution of the group as a collective subject comes about in a rapid moment of fusion.

However, I would add that there is a long series of events that prepare for this development in a small group:

- People realise that their belonging to the group is no longer under discussion.
- They become more inclined to put themselves at risk.
- They see the therapist as being less rigid and distant, and more human and vulnerable.

Fusion of the group

Sartre sees the group not as a structure but as a process, as the dialectic mediator between the isolated individual, alienated by inertia and seriality, experimenting with the kind of human relationship in which every member is undifferentiated and replaceable by another, and a society which is crystallised into rigid institutions. The isolated individual, in fact, is neither able to make his voice heard by society, nor to counteract or modify nature.

A second essential feature of Sartre's argument is his recognition that the individual can be isolated even when he is not alone; for example, people waiting at a bus stop experience a common situation, the discomfort is the same, but they do not communicate. They are isolated.

According to Sartre the fusion of the group leads individuals to emerge from isolation, alienation and impotence. Emerging from passivity, a man joins a group, or together with others forms a group, which acts upon reality. He is no longer a man facing the world alone, but he is part of a small group through which he can adapt or else modify reality.

In overcoming seriality individuals establish a relationship of reciprocity. 'Reciprocity is the relationship according to which every individual, for the other, is himself' (see Aebischer and Oberle 1990, pp.106–107; Anzieu 1988, p.XI; Rosenfeld 1988, pp.4 and 5).

- They lose their dependence on and fear of the therapist; while previously they waited before intervening (for approval, disapproval, or salvation), now there are long periods in which the group almost forgets him.

- They no longer turn only to the analyst, but try to locate their personal thoughts and questions within the group field, sometimes succeeding in inserting them into the collective functioning and other times not (see De Risio 1986; Puget *et al.* 1991).

From the point of view of technique it is important to note that the passage from one phase to another of the group often coincides with a change in role for those taking part. In a group which I led, for example, one person who in the initial part of group work (the Emerging state) had played the part of welcomer, encourager and co-ordinater of the group, so much so that she had been jokingly called 'the group's mum', took on a completely different role when we got to the Fraternal Community phase. Her new role in the group was marked by a long period of silence after which she re-emerged in a role that was much more problematic and less 'efficient'.

The Fraternal Community stage

As I mentioned before, when the stage which I have just described is reached it is characterised by the appearance on the scene of a collective subject.

Concerning this, I should like to emphasise that the active emergence of the group as a collective subject (in Freud's terms, a Fraternal Community or Clan) introduces one of the most interesting operative possibilities of the group setting (the presence of several people) which I mentioned in the Introduction (see De Simone 1981). The traditional (couple) setting requires the analyst and analysand to be alone in the consulting room and any other presences are phantasies evoked by the imaginative force of speech. In the group setting, on the contrary, the presence of others, i.e. the group members who are taking part in the analytic work, is essential. This difference is relevant both at the level of phantasy and in the way it affects the progress of analytic work. More precisely, the presence of several people both with regard to phantasy and to analytic work is evident in two forms: the 'co-members' and the 'Fraternal Community'. The first form (co-members) corresponds to the presence of the other members as individuals, towards whom every participant may possibly have feelings of protection, admiration, jealousy, rivalry and envy. The second form (Fraternal Community) corresponds to the members as components of a whole of which all members are a part and which has particular characteristics and functions.

The nucleus of the new fundamental law on which the group as a Fraternal Community is founded, and which governs relationships within it, is the fact that the participants realise that they have a right with respect to the group. The holder of this right is not one single person, but every individual in so far as he is a part of the Fraternal Community. In this regard L. Levy Bruehl (1922, pp.101, 122, 131 and 228) made a useful observation: 'Primitives do not understand that the earth is subject to individual ownership. The earth in reality belongs – in the absolute sense – to the whole social group, that is to say to all the living and the dead together.'

Technique

P. Privat and J.B. Chapelier, and Privat, J. and Privat, P. (1987; 1987) declare that the group can come to life and take on a structure only if the therapist plays an active part, but that, at other times, he needs to keep his distance from group life if he is to carry out his function.

I agree wholeheartedly with this declaration. A group therapist must understand when the Fraternal Community stage is maturing in the group, and realise when he needs to step back, to take a back seat, and then later to find a way of intervening which will respect the functioning of the group as a collective subject.

CHAPTER 4

The Group's Common Space

In the two preceding chapters I have outlined corresponding moments in the history of the group: (the Emerging state and the stage of the group as a collective subject or Fraternal Community); I should like now to consider the creation of the group's common space. The creation of such a space corresponds to the time of leaving the Emerging state and reaching the stage of the group as a collective subject. The group's common space, in fact, provides an instrument essential to making possible collective forms of thought, and counteracts the experiences of depersonalisation which are characteristic of a newly emerging group.

The creation of space-time

What do we mean when we talk about the common space which is created within the group? I believe that such a space is not actually materially measurable, that it does not correspond to a territory which can be described or travelled through, that it does not coincide with the 'geographic' or organisational boundaries of the group, but that it is a mental and relational space (see Figa Talamanca 1991; Marinelli 1991; Siracusano 1986). Its dimensions are those of the capacity for thought acquired by the group members. From this viewpoint, Arendt (1963) has given us a coherent definition, in which the term 'space' refers not to a territory, but to the space existing between individuals forming a group, that is to say individuals bound one to another (but at the same time separated and protected) by the many things which they have in common. The common space of the group members is therefore closely linked to their feeling of belonging and with a distinction between what the group is and what it is not. J. Lotman clarifies this aspect of the definition of space. According to him, the cultural and social area of a group is distinguished from the exterior by a sort of boundary. The interior is experienced by those belonging to the group, and is essentially seen as being structured; while the exterior is perceived as being unstructured.

Lotman's idea can be represented schematically: the common space, the area of belonging is IN. IN, from the point of view of a member of the group, tends to be identified with the concept of order, and is in polarity with EXT, the non-group or chaos. Belonging to IN means existing. Being expelled from it means not existing, finishing up in the non-real, the indefinite.

Mental skin

An important part in the setting up of group boundaries is played by the members transfering their 'mental skin' function to the group. In other words, from a certain point onwards in the vicissitudes of the group, the boundary function is no longer entrusted to single individuals, but is taken over, to a great extent, by the group. A visual image of this kind of phenomenon is given in certain documentary films involving street demonstrations, where it can be seen how the advance of the first ranks causes the ones behind to close up. On the other hand, if the front ranks are seen to yield the whole group may break up and take flight.

Although this image refers to a mass and not to a small group, it gives an effective idea of the dimension of the sensorial and bodily phenomena to which I am referring (see Corrao 1986, p.20; Dell'Anna 1993).

The transfer of the function of boundary from the individual to the group as a whole and the creation of the group's common space are favoured by some of the participants' sensorial, emotive and mental experiences in the course of the sessions. I shall now indicate a few of them.

- The physical impression that when people are seated in a circle they define a space.

- The perception that some sensations – in particular, those of excitement, fear or tension – have group rather than individual rhythms: as though the group as a whole was regulating or not managing to regulate them.

- The realisation that thoughts and emotions can circulate in a wider context than the one which the members assign to their own experiences when they think individually (see Americo 1983, pp.91–97; Ruberti 1990, pp.21–28).

I shall bring this chapter to a close with a few words by D. Anzieu (1981) which effectively sum up the argument. According to Anzieu, a group is a casing which holds individuals together. Until this casing is put in place we are talking about a human aggregate, not a group.

A casing which holds together thoughts, words and actions enables the group to build up an internal space. This gives a feeling of liberty and guarantees that exchanges will continue within the group. The group has its own temporality, which includes a past from which the group derives its origins, and a future in which it plans to pursue its aims.

CHAPTER 5

Genius Loci

The division between the IN and EXT of the group, described by J. Lotman (1978), which I spoke of in the last chapter, can be more or less rigid. The degree of rigidity of this boundary determines whether the members feel that the experience of the small analytic group is completely separate from everyday life, or distinct but not in opposition. In turn, the rigidity of the boundary depends on the identity of the group. The more a group has built up an identity which is not based on opposition to the external world, the more flexible and permeable the boundary is. As W. Benjamin says (1931): 'the threshold must be clearly distinguished from the boundary. In the word threshold we include change, passage, tides'.

The spirit of the place

The rigidity of the group boundary and the sense of identity of its members can be related to a function which I call 'the function of the group's Genius loci'. I should like to present this function with a mythological allusion.

The Greeks and Romans connected places with a divinity: the Genius loci.

Every fountain, every mountain, had a divine guardian.

If the place were to remain intact and out of reach of their enemies, the deity had to live there constantly. As a consequence, the gods' tranquillity was not to be disturbed.

In fact, the Genius loci had a special relationship with the harmony of the place. It governed relationships between the various elements: water, winds, vegetation, buildings, etc. It got irritated if the characteristics and special qualities of the place were altered by actions and movements against its nature. (see Cinti 1989, p.134)

Architects now call on the expression Genius loci to explain why it would not be appropriate to build Alpine chalets (or eight-storey skyscrapers) on the coasts of

Sicily or Calabria. Man-made constructions have to be in harmony with the Genius loci, with the spirit of the place and with the landscape. The Genius loci is therefore something which comes from nature and the environment and then includes man-made elements. The task of the Genius loci in the small analytic group is to animate or reanimate the identity of the group, to link the progress of the group to its emotive basis.

What is more, the Genius loci also has the task of preventing the group from becoming sclerotic or excessively institutionalised, and in addition, of avoiding lacerations and wounds in the syncretic identity of the members, while at the same time permitting the group situation to evolve.

Syncretic sociality

Syncretic sociality is not very evolved, it is basic, and founded on feelings and experiences that are difficult to put into words. It is the basis of the syncretic identity of the group members. Bleger writes (1967a, pp.511–512):

> In all groups there exists another identity [different from evolved identity and this identity]. This is sometimes the only one, or the only one which can be achieved in that group; it is a very special identity which we can call syncretic group identity, and which depends, not on integration, interaction or rules at an evolved level, but on socialisation where there are no such limits. None of those we see, from a naturalistic point of view, as subjects, individuals or persons, possess an identity as such; their identity is in their belonging to the group.

The non-verbal syncretic level and the evolved level of the relationship are not separable. On the contrary, they are strongly interdependent. Bleger gives an effective illustration of this point:

> In a room a mother may be reading, watching the television or busy cooking. In the same room her son is busy playing on his own. If we were to consider the level of interaction, we would see no communication between these two people; they are not speaking to each other or looking at each other; each is acting independently, in isolation, and we might say that there is no interaction or that they are not in communication. This is true if we only consider the interaction level. But, let's continue with our example. The mother suddenly leaves what she is doing and goes out of the room; the child immediately stops playing and runs out to be near her. We now realise that when the mother and child were each busy with a different task, without speaking to each other or communicating at an interaction level, there was still a deep-seated non-verbal bond between them, which had no need of words, which, on the contrary, would have been disturbed by words. In other terms, when there is no interaction and they are not even looking at each other or speaking to each other, syncretic sociality is present. The two people we had considered isolated from a naturalistic point of view, were in a state of fusion and not distinction. (1967a, pp.511–513)

If there is any attack on syncretic sociality, the result is a seriously disturbed situation. Moreover, attacks of this kind often lead to sub-group clashes. Unyielding opposing sub-groups are created not so much because there are differing opinions as because there is an identical wound in their syncretic identity, which each sub-group can feel but denies having received. Each feels that something serious and fundamental has happened, something which touches it closely. A certain image of the group has been damaged. A certain understanding of sociality has been offended. Something which provided a bridge enabling members to identify themselves with the group has been changed. Each sub-group blames the other sub-group for the damage and deals with it as an internal struggle. Bion (1961, pp.38–39) expresses supplementary ideas to those I have just illustrated. He affirms in fact that the schism (the sub-division of a group into opposing sub-groups) occurs when a push towards progress is seen as a risk to the primitive mentality of this same group. Bion observes that the two opposed sub-groups are not one a supporter of the 'rational group' and the other a supporter of the 'primitive group', but that both tend to bring to a halt what is felt to be a catastrophic overall change for the group. In other words, if progress is too rapid it generates conflict to the extent of harming sociality and syncretic identity (see Grinberg, Tabak and De Bianchedi 1972).

Group identity

After this long digression aimed at illustrating the notion of syncretic sociality and its link with an internal struggle which may arise in the group, I should like to return to the Genius loci.

As I said, the Genius loci takes on the task of preserving group identity. This saves the group from having to resort to the idea of an enemy or of a rigid boundary between internal and external in order to maintain and confirm its own identity. The rigidity of group boundaries is a sign of a failure (or lack) of this aspect of the Genius loci function, where the group, to defend its own coherence, has to resort to a very large extent to its members' archaic (ethological) ability to set up the boundaries of a territory. In this case the boundary is no longer a membrane, but a barrier. The weaving activity of the Genius loci is internal and secret. Internal and secret because it goes on within its own identity. The analyst must understand and follow up the activity of the Genius loci, but he must not make it the object of interpretations. Nor is it appropriate that the person who most embodies it should be explicitly indicated. This identification may, in fact, obstruct rather than facilitate the development of the function.

Genius loci and the operative therapist

In chapter 11 I shall quote a passage taken from Virginia Woolf, in which she depicts the figure of a woman who functions as a Genius loci for a group made up of friends and family. I now intend to show how the figure of the Genius loci and that of the group therapist do not coincide. The therapist in the work-group is a 'responsible operator'. The Genius loci is a figure of emotional relevance. The operative leader of the analytic group deals with truth and knowledge, and the Genius loci with the emotive heritage of the group, its vitality and freshness. The leader's function is to direct the group in carrying out its task. The function of the Genius loci is to find ways of staying together, ways which will activate the 'group spirit'. This means choosing – according to the moment and its appropriateness – thoughtfulness, happiness or pain.

The Genius loci is not usually the group's analyst. To be able to operate effectively, the Genius loci must be seen to be a figure on a par with the members of the group. The therapist's position does not permit him to take on this role. He is the pole of intense projections and expectations, he is a somewhat idealised figure, or at least he coincides with an idealised aspect of the group, that is to say, psychoanalysis (see Ferruta 1992).

The Genius loci and the group therapist usually work side by side. Sometimes, however, they may be momentarily in opposition. The activation of the 'group spirit' sometimes causes disorder. At times confusion and chaos may occur. These moments are tolerated and actually promoted by the Genius loci, while they may cause suffering and anguish in the operative group therapist who is weighed down by responsibility for the efficiency and good image of the group.

PART 3
The Field

In the previous section I described how the group is set up as a unit during the Emerging stage and then how, in the Fraternal Community stage, it begins to function as a subject capable of thought. In developing this argument I took into special account the formation of a group boundary and the contemporaneous phenomenon of the creation of the group's common space. The concept of the field, which I shall present in this chapter, is a deepening and extending of the group's common space. To be more precise, it is the convergence of my observations about the creation of the group's common space and those relating to the transpersonal phenomena (atmosphere of the group, medium, effects of basic assumptions and collective mentality) which I spoke about in the first chapter.

The concept of semiosphere – which I shall illustrate next – again starts off from the idea of the group's common space, and its aim is to examine one of its functions: that of supporting the thought of the group and of its members.

CHAPTER 6

The Field

The concept of field – based on contributions from various psychoanalysts and group therapists – involves different levels of meaning. As a result of this stratification process several rather disparate 'sense nuclei' co-exist in this notion. For my part I shall not even attempt to propose a univocal (or unitary) view of the idea. Any effort in this direction, in fact, would necessarily involve ignoring a series of contributions of considerable theoretical interest with corresponding clinical practice. My approach is aimed more at reconciling the various nuclei and models.

In the first part of the chapter I shall examine two field models, which emphasise its spatial dimensions. I will refer to M. and W. Baranger's bi-personal concept of the field and to the idea of the field as a 'transpersonal container'. Under this heading I can gather a series of hypotheses advanced by J. Bleger, A. Correale and P. Perrotti. Of course, not all the authors I have just mentioned speak explicitly about the field, but I do believe that their observations can be used to give substance to the concept.

In the second part of the chapter I shall consider the possibility of seeing the field as a shared mental state. My argument stems from one of W.R. Bion's observations. Considering the field as a mental state brings this notion close to those of the medium and of primitive mentality which I illustrated both in 'Historical Notes' and in Chapter 1.

Finally, in the third part of this chapter, I shall illustrate a few elements which specifically characterise the notion of field, proposing the concepts of synchrony and interdependence.

Field, space, setting

In discussions between group therapists – which take place for example in supervisions and seminars – the terms 'field' and 'group space' are often used as synonyms. This informal and colloquial use is probably a reflection of the impact which the notion of the bi-personal field has had on analysts and group therapists.

The concept of the bi-personal field has been set down by M. and W. Baranger. These two Franco-Argentinian psychoanalysts begin by drawing attention to the inevitable involvement of the psychoanalyst as co-protagonist of the analytic experience, and they come to the conclusion that psychoanalyst and patient form an inextricably linked and complementary couple, taking part in the same dynamic process.

Their second affirmation is much more innovative. They say that the patient-therapist dyad generates a field and is included in the field which it produces. W. and M. Baranger then differentiate the field from the two personalities involved in the relationship. The bi-personal field cannot be considered the sum of the two internal psychic situations, since it is something which is created between the two, within the unity which they constitute at the time of the session. The bi-personal field is moreover something which is very different from what either of the two is, considered separately. Take for example the situation of a married couple where they create a field of quarrelling. The quarrelling exists independently of the two individuals' will and occurs each time these two people are together. It cannot be attributed to either of them since it somehow goes beyond their relationship and its vicissitudes. The analytic couple, according to M. and W. Baranger, originates something which is like a third party, i.e. a field, which has its own qualities and dynamics which are independent of the two individuals involved in the relationship.

M. and W. Baranger further develop their model by indicating that the field has three levels of structure. The first is the setting, the second the verbal transaction which takes place in the session, the third is the bi-personal unconscious phantasy. What is specific to the analytic experience is the possibility of making contact with this phantasy and therefore with the latent structure of the field.

Finally, the Barangers emphasise the importance of the concept of field in analytic work. The analytic situation has its own spatial and temporal structure, and is governed by fixed dynamics and forces; it possesses its own laws of development and general and particular objectives. It is this field, M. and W. Baranger conclude, that is our immediate and specific source of information. The notion of a bi-personal field has been worked out with reference to the classic (dual) analytic situation, but it can be usefully extended to include the group analytic situation. In this case we speak of a multi-personal field. In the concept of the multi-personal field attention is turned to the way in which the group members and the analyst contribute to the maintenance of the group field and how they are conditioned by it.

In addition, this notion leads us to consider a technical problem relating to the organisation of the group. A series of 'responses' must potentially be present and ready ('stationed') in the shared situation (in the multi-personal field) so that interaction can be delicately regulated. For example, if the *acting* of one of the group participants should lead to an abrupt intervention by the analyst, that would mean that the multi-personal field had not been smoothed out and harmonised in advance in its various aspects (space–time structure, setting, verbal transaction) in such a way as to be sure of a ready (spontaneous) response, which can be used for the understanding and working through of what has now been made evident by this impulsive *acting*.

The concept of 'bi-personal unconscious phantasy' deserves separate treatment. As we have seen, this constitutes the third level of structuring of the 'multi-personal field'. First of all, I should like to explain that the notion of 'bi--personal unconscious phantasy' cannot be simply reduced to the conception of 'unconscious phantasy' classically formulated, (for example, by S. Isaacs), as the expression of the life of an individual's instincts. Bi-personal or multi-personal unconscious phantasy is in fact made up of a puzzle of projective identifications which involves, to a varying extent, both the members of the group and the analyst. On the other hand, it is possible to closely compare the idea of bi-personal unconscious phantasy and above all that of multi-personal unconscious phantasy with the idea of primitive mentality (basic assumptions) (Baranger and Baranger 1961–1962).

In *Experiences in Groups* (1961) Bion puts forward the hypothesis that primitive mentality is a common reservoir into which the contributions of all the members of the group flow, and in which the impulses and desires these contributions contain can be gratified.

If we then bear in mind that Madeleine and Willy Baranger's unconscious phantasy is an accumulation of projective identifications, we will notice a few points of contact between the two notions. These points mainly consist of the idea of a collective depository and of the use of projective identification. In *A Theory of Thought* (1962, pp.180–181) Bion in fact speaks about the development of social capacity, basing this on a capacity to communicate. This, in turn, has its basis in the use of 'realistic projective identification' (see Bezoari and Ferro 1991, pp.8–9; Sarno 1982 and 1983).

The field as transpersonal depository

One way of understanding the field, to a certain extent similar to that of M. and W. Baranger, is to consider it as a special trans-personal pool of feelings, emotions and ideas present in the session and more generally in the group. It is a transpersonal pool, in the sense that it is beyond individuals and does not correspond to their relationships, and yet conditions both individuals and relationships (Di Trapani *et al*. 1994).

A. Correale, who dwells on the notion of the field as a pool, states that the field must be seen more as a fluid situation than as a structured one, as a situation in constant movement, to which the individuals belonging to a certain group contribute, but which at the same time conditions them.

He describes the field as a complex and mobile amalgamation in which various elements converge. The field (as a pool) is for individual members either a place which is different and distinct from themselves, in which they can keep feelings and tensions separate, or at the same time an extension of themselves. For a clearer description of the elements which compose this amalgamation, Correale distinguishes an 'actual field' and a 'historical field'. The 'historical field' (historical memory) of the group is constantly kept up to date and conditions the actual field (the field present at a given time in the group).

Actual field and historical field

The actual field (here-and-now field) is: 'the result of the combination of the images, thoughts [phantasies], representations [deposited in the group], but also the affects, instincts, emotions and feelings present and active in the group at a given moment'.

An indication of what the here-and-now field is comes from the atmosphere which prevails in the session, an atmosphere which immediately draws the attention of anyone entering a group for the first time, and expresses in an almost tactile and physical way the moment the group is experiencing.

However, the group field (on the whole) is, at the same time, also the result of the contribution of the historical field. That is to say, of 'a slow depositing of affective relationships, of imagined, representative and emotive vicissitudes. This deposit enriches and at the same time weighs down on the life of the group, forming its memory, which is largely unaware, partly propulsive, partly inhibiting and blocking' (Correale 1992).

P. Perrotti does not speak explicitly about the field, but more in general about the group. However, what he says can be related to the argument I am developing. Perrotti suggests that the group is a place in which group members can deposit not only feelings, emotions and affects, but also parts of themselves that they wish to get rid of. An active 'capture' of these refused elements by the group would correspond to a 'deposit' by its members. Perrotti writes (1983): 'The group [conversely] would pick up individuals' split parts and favour the formation of psychotic cysts which would be seen as being split from the normal parts of the personality.'

J. Bleger, too, does not use the exact term 'field', but 'setting'. However I believe I can use his contributions as well. According to Bleger, the deposit of the psychotic aspects of the personality takes place in those dimensions of the setting (the room, the timetable, the analyst's attitude) which are most stable in time (setting-institution). Bleger observes that under normal conditions the bond between the patient in analysis and the setting (in which he has deposited the psychotic aspects of his identities) is silent. On the other hand, the patient may behave in a completely unexpected way compared to past experience, when there is a break or the risk of a break in the setting and therefore in the relationship with the analytic situation. Bleger (1967a) observes on this point 'it has always seemed to me both surprising and fascinating to note...how the patient can be upset and become violent, for example, by a difference of a few minutes at the beginning or the end of a session'. The reason for these violent outbursts of rage becomes comprehensible if we advance the hypothesis that the patient has 'deposited' the psychotic aspects of his identity in the setting-institution, imagining that they were completely under control, just as if it were one of his arms. Even a small variation in the setting-institution makes him realise that this container is not a part of him, that he is not in complete control of it.

At this point he is seized by panic, feels unprotected, and loses the ability to maintain coherence in his thoughts and emotions.

Bleger also offers another observation which is important for the development of the notion of the field as a container. He points out how patients not only deposit in the setting (in the field) the psychotic parts of their identity, but also very vital and essential aspects of themselves. Bleger (1967a, pp.511–513) says that in particular the deposit may concern the *non-changing* aspects of identity. The *non-changing* part of the identity, in turn, is a source of security for a more mature identity.

I shall bring to an end this part of the argument regarding the field by pointing out that thinking of the field as a transpersonal container explains the fact that a problem posed by one of the participants, for example, during one of the first sessions, may apparently not be received by the other members and instead get an 'unexpected' response much later on.

The model of the field as a transpersonal container in fact makes possible the hypothesis that the problem together with various and successive 'drafts' of responses are deposited in the field until the moment when it is possible to express them.

The mental state-field

A different line of theoretical development indicates the field as being a mental state. By mental state I do not simply mean an idea, but a complex system of phantasies, emotions and ideas which are all linked together.

There are two different viewpoints from which we can consider the definition of the field as a mental state. The first can be presented by a note by W.R. Bion (1987, pp.139–141).

Speaking of analytic work with 'serious' and borderline patients (patients on the borderline between a neurotic and a psychotic personality), he makes an observation which is summed up as follows:

> Borderline patients are in a position to notice when the analyst turns his mind away from them, even for a few seconds; it is as though a field were established, supported by the analyst's attention, and the patient can perceive his slightest lowering of intensity or shortest interruptions; these patients, in fact, depend on being thought of by the analyst in order to maintain a certain coherence in themselves.

The mental state-field at which Bion hints when speaking of borderline patients is relatively neutral from the point of view of the emotions. The analyst's attention is its basic dimension. Its function is to maintain the possibility of relationships and thought in the patient in analysis. This is also true of the group. For example, whether anyone speaking in public can present a well-ordered argument depends largely on the attention with which his speech is followed. Other phenomena of the same type are difficult to explain in words, but we have all noticed them frequently. If someone is in a room, and another person is watching him from behind, the first person feels he is being watched and turns round. It is difficult to say what has happened, but there have been small changes, minute maybe muscular signals or other tensions, which show a variation in the field through which the person who is being watched knows that something has changed. I can clarify my opinion on this first definition of the field notion as a mental state by saying that it is a relatively neutral medium from the emotive point of view. It is more of a basic support. Other fields, other collective mental states, have strong emotive connotations. A clinical example will illustrate this.

> In the course of a session of a group of ex-drug addicts and drug addicts being treated with methadone, they talk about the difficulty (or rather the impossibility) of 'getting high' without resorting to substances like heroin, cocaine and alcohol.
>
> At the following session, one of the members, Lorenzo, comes to the group after taking heroin. He speaks at length and very intensely, relating a series of dramatic and paradoxical episodes and alternating these with the expression of his needs and desires.
>
> Lorenzo's story and his way of speaking activates a 'field' in the group which corresponds to the mental state of 'being on a high', the absence of which the members of the group had been complaining of. (This group was led by Dr Teresa Centro, at the LSU drug addiction service of Naples-Ponticelli.)

Like the phenomena of the emerging stage of the group, the mental state-field necessarily involves all the members of a certain group; it also influences their way of perceiving and expressing thoughts and feelings. For example, a feeling of fear experienced by one of the participants may be alleviated or, on the contrary, accentuated, when it is immersed in the mental state-field of the group.

It is calmed if the field is receptive, and becomes more acute if the field is tense and dominated by anxiety.

Another important characteristic of some forms of 'mental state-field' is the ability to exist over and above spatial limits: over and above the apparent limits of the Maginot line between the two opposing military camps, the French and the German, the mental field (feelings of fear, hate, hope, desire to fraternise and to return home) was one and the same.

Neither is a mental state-field limited by time. For example, a 'field of hate' may appear at completely different times from the one in which it originated, using people who are drawn into passions and events which dominate them in order to emerge, just like a virus does with living cells. An illustration is given by L. Borges in 'Brodie's Manuscript' (1970).

> The story is seen through the eyes of a child who is attentive yet at the same time detached. The events are suspended in a dreamlike legendary time. The protagonists are now dead and the narrator himself is old.

> About twelve people have met for an *asado* in a villa outside the town. They are all young people between twenty and thirty. After dinner a guitar is played, coffee and cigars are handed round and time passes slowly. One of the guests suggests to another a two-handed game of poker. The sensation is one of a possible dramatic development. One of those present tries in vain to prevent it.

> During the card game the child goes away to explore the house and gets lost in the darkness. The host finds him and takes him to look at a glass case where some knives are displayed which are famous because in the past they had been used by bandits. His explanation is interrupted by angry voices.

> A quarrel has broken out in the next room. One of the guests, Uriarte, repeatedly accuses another, Duncan, of cheating. Duncan finally reacts and punches him. One of the guests remarks that there is no lack of weapons. The glass case is opened. Uriarte chooses a weapon with a U-shaped hilt, Duncan a knife with a wooden handle and the figure of a little tree on the blade.

> Duncan and Uriarte show an unusual and unexpected mastery in using knives. The fight becomes bloody; no one dares intervene. Duncan is mortally wounded. All those present agree to call it a regular duel, and not to mention what has really happened. The child is extremely shocked by what he has seen.

> He keeps the secret for a long time. Many years later, by that time a man, he meets a friend, a police official, an expert in adventurers, criminals and murders. Borges' friend is able to reconstruct the identities of the former owners of the two knives. They were two famous knife-throwers. They had the same name. They hated each other. They had continued to look for each other throughout

their lives, but never managed to meet. Borges ends the story with these words: 'Maneco Uriarte did not kill Duncan; the weapons, not the men, were fighting.

'They had slept side by side in the glass case until hands had awoken them... They had sought each other for a long time... Human bitterness slept and waited within their metal.'

I shall not linger any longer over the a-spatial and a-temporal characteristics of collective field-mental states; I shall return to this subject in Chapter 18, which is devoted to the transpersonal diffusion of phantasies and mental states. I want now to begin the last part of my explanation of the notion of the field, dealing with synchronicity and interdependence.

Synchronicity

I shall begin with a definition: the field can be considered, besides being a transpersonal container and a mental state, as a system of synchronicity and inter-dependence. This definition helps in establishing a distinction between the notion of the field and that of the common space of the group, which considers above all the aspect of limit of the group (see La Forgia 1992).

The optics of synchronicity considers feelings, ideas, facts, which happen in the group, as copresent, whether they belong to the present or the past, or whether they are simply expectations or fears for the future. To assume the vertex of synchronicity means, then, to operate a strong compression of temporal per-spectives: time is condensed into 'here and now'. The adoption of a particular method of thought also corresponds to the temporal perspective I have indicated: a thought which does not separate, choose, isolate and classify, but takes on the whole of present events, as though expressing a meaning. For example, if in a group a person comes in and begins to cough and then stands up; another mem-ber talks about the need to sacrifice oneself, to put oneself in second place; a third person speaks of the problems he had when his brothers were born; all these ele-ments should be considered as capable of expressing a comprehensive meaning. On this subject C.G. Jung (1948, pp.13–14) writes:

> This assumption implies a strange principle which I have called synchronicity, a concept which formulates a point of view diametrically opposed to causality... This latter [shows] how events evolve one from the other, while synchronicity considers the coincidence of events in space and time as meaning something more than a mere chance, that is to say a particular interdependence of events that are objective from each other, as between them and the subjective (psychic) conditions of the observer or observers...

> As causality explains the sequence of events...synchronicity explains their co-incidence. The causal point of view tells us a dramatic story of the way in which D came into existence; originating from C who existed before D, and C in his turn had a father who was B, etc. The synchronistic view, for its part, tries to

produce an equally significant picture of the coincidence: how does it happen that A, B, C, D etc. all appear at the same moment and in the same place?

Interdependence

The elements which form a field are linked by synchronicity. They are also interdependent. The link of interdependence is different, more complex but equally strong or stronger than a link of similarity. The elements of the field are not necessarily similar to each other, but once a link of interdependence is established it may be stronger than a link based on similarity. After a certain configuration of the field is established, if one of the elements is modified, all are modified. By the effect of the relationship of interdependence, a change of state of any part or fraction of the elements which take part in the field influences the state of all the others (see Lewin, 1936, pp.53–54; 1948, p.125).

Interdependence is the expression of a relationship which is established or establishes itself between the elements, not only 'horizontally' but also between different levels of experience of the members of the group. On the other hand, the field – which is shaped by the choices of relationship operated on these elements – progressively becomes an attractor, a container of other thoughts and feelings, a place of transformation and change (see Corrente 1992, pp.57–60; Luhmann 1980, pp.236–249; Pribram 1991, p.11; Romano 1986, pp.40–41).

Interdependence is a link which can be established by means of a choice. This point has been brought out by Bion when he speaks of the oscillation of PsD, that is the oscillation between dispersion and individuation and the activity of an ordinating principle (a chosen fact, a significant configuration) which takes upon itself to propose and evaluate a link between the elements which were first dispersed. It is interesting to reflect on this suggestion in terms of 'fact' or 'chosen fact'. If a certain series of elements are present at the same time – for example overcrowding, violence, opposed ideological pressure, rage – we may soon find ourselves facing a fact (a revolt, a civil war). If a series of 'chatter' is circulated without anyone evaluating it or taking a stand, the diverse chatter becomes 'gossip', autonomous and uncontrollable. If a choice is not made, if no responsibility is assumed for the significance implicit in that certain series of elements present in the small group, these elements will 'come to an agreement' on their own and we shall next find ourselves facing a fact, something produced by these elements but from which the thinking subject or subjects are in some way excluded. To establish a meaning, a relationship of interdependence between the elements, implies evaluating, choosing and assuming responsibility. Equally, I believe, within the group there may be a series of confused elements (for example: discomfort, an atmosphere of stagnation, failed attempts to advance). There is the possibility that someone will assume the task of suggesting a sense, selecting elements and thus giving a form to the field. But maybe this will not happen, and then these elements interact and present themselves as a 'given field' which the members find themselves faced with.

Concluding considerations

As I have already said when introducing this chapter, I shall not try to operate a synthesis between the different nuclei of meaning which join to form the idea of the field; I shall limit myself only to indicating a few possible links.

An intersection between the multi-personal field which has been described by M. and W. Baranger and the field as a system of synchronicity and interdependence may be pinpointed by reflecting on that part of M. and W. Baranger's definition which indicates that the multi-personal field is directed according to lines of force and fixed dynamics, and has its own laws of development. This conception of the field, in fact, can easily be integrated with the idea that the field is governed by the laws of synchronicity and interdependence.

A relationship between the field as a 'transpersonal container' and 'field-mental state' may be established by paying particular attention to the 'historical field'. In the last book of I. Metter (1992, p.127), there is a fine image. Metter writes that in certain environments – public lavatories, breweries, stations – an odour has been deposited, so specific and characteristic that even though the rooms have been thoroughly aired, we continue to perceive that this odour has pervaded the environment. Similarly, going into certain groups, we feel, for example, a sense of longstanding rancour, or of gloom and boredom which cannot be removed. Going into other groups, we have a sense of mental openness and lightness. If the group produces certain 'mental fields', these can permeate what Correale has defined as 'historical field', giving origin to a quality of culture, of belonging to this certain group, which cannot easily be modified and transformed.

CHAPTER 7

Self-Representation and Semiosphere

When I spoke about the group's common space in Chapter 4, I dealt with the boundary which the group establishes with the external world. I should like to take up the argument again, underlining how, as the group acquires a more solid identity, right from the Fraternal Community stage, the boundary of the group with the outside world loses relevance and the group turns inwards. In more explicit terms: the participants make an effort to represent and give sense to what is 'within' the group. The group could then be described as being like certain Mediterranean houses, which have only a few small windows facing outwards, while internally they open on to a shady and lively courtyard.

Having clarified the general theme, I shall give a few indications of how I have sub-divided it. In the first part of the chapter I shall illustrate a few ideas of various authors which are quite close to the theme I intend to tackle. My aim is to create a background of propositions and suggestions against which the subject can be placed.

I shall then introduce the concept of 'self-representation', recalling some of Lotman's studies, and I shall illustrate one of the analytic group's systems of self-representation, i.e. the dream. Finally, in the last part of the chapter, I shall link up the notion of self-representation with the setting, and introduce the notion of semiosphere.

I should like to anticipate a first definition of semiosphere. The semiosphere is the ambit for determining the sense of what happens in the group and includes all the functions which preside in it. These functions are self-representation, the γ-functions, group associative chains and mimesis. In the real life of the analytic group these functions or systems do not exist in an isolated condition. Their division into separate parts is only a heuristic necessity. Taken one by one, none of these parts is really able to function, doing so only if immersed in a semeiotic continuum full of formations of different types placed at various levels of organisation. I shall call semiosphere the body of these systems for working out sense and the continuum of which they are part. (see Lotman 1985, p.56)

Self-representation

Ideas which may be closely compared to the concept of self-representation have already been used by various authors in connection with the group. The expression 'self-centred group', for example, indicates a reflection of the group about itself (see Borgogno 1977).

In the Northfield experiment, Bion tried to create an operative situation in which everyone could see himself and the group, as though looking into a building with glass walls.

K. Lewin and his collaborators speak of supplying 'feedback' to group members on the progress of the dynamics in which they are involved.

Feedback

In 1946, Kurt Lewin, at that time director of the Research Center for Group Dynamics at the MIT, was requested by the educational psychologist Leland Bradford to lead, with his research team, a residential 'information' seminar for 65 teachers from the state of Maine. During pauses in their seminar work, the 'leaders' were accustomed to discussing among themselves the efficacy of lessons and lectures, the reactions of teachers who were taking part, how the seminar was going and its evolution. One evening, during a meeting, the animators were 'taken by surprise' by some seminar participants requesting to attend. Lewin agreed, and Zander, Lippit and Bradford, his colleagues in the working team, had no objections. The participants were very interested in what they heard in this informal meeting, finding that observations on their behaviour in the group were much more interesting and stimulating than the lectures they attended during the day and the follow-up discussions. They asked if they could continue to take part in the meetings, and also devote part of their seminar work to reflection on group interaction and on the attitudes of each of them in the course of the seminar. In this way the principle of giving back to the group, through feedback, an image of its behaviour was determined (see Carli 1993).

S.H. Foulkes (1964, p.104) suggests comparing group analysis to psychodrama. In particular he draws attention to the dramatic nature of the communications which take place during the session. Alongside the dramatic character of communications, there are two other analogies between psychodrama and group analysis which can be noted. The first regards the dual role of actor and participating audience which is played both by participants in a psychodrama and by members of an analytic group. The second regards a characteristic which, at certain times, is taken on by the 'common space' of the group members. This space, in fact, becomes a sort of imaginary stage on which the participants' phantasies are performed. However, it is necessary to underline a few substantial differences: in group analysis, movements and gestures as means of expression are relinquished (words become more important), and the 'common space' of the group is not a real, but a mental stage.

Psychodrama

In Jacob Moreno's psychodrama (1948) those participating in the group are used both as the theatrical company and as the audience, in order to explore individual problems, through their re-actualisation and staging. In some specialised centres or institutions a platform is raised, to serve as a stage on which the group members in turn present their problems. The patient chosen to be the lead selects his assistants from among the other members of the group, and helps them to play the part assigned to them, by describing in great detail the scene he wants to perform.

From time to time the therapist-producer may give instructions to one of the participants who is in the audience to take on the lead role (reversal of the roles of 'actors' and 'audience'). In this way, in the discussion which follows the performance, several people are able to express their opinion, based on direct experience (see Brown and Pedder 1991, pp.119 and 169–70).

Cinema, theatre, literature

References to K. Lewin's T-group and J. Moreno's psychodrama are useful as a general evocative background. I shall try now to put the argument more precisely. I will attempt to show that the central problem posed by the idea of self-representation in the small group is to clarify how the level of communication refers back to the deeper phantasies of the group members. Some indications of J. Lotman (1985, pp.55–76) are particularly useful in dealing with this problem.

Lotman shows how the behaviour and even the feelings, which people belonging to a certain society and a certain culture experience in their everyday life, are in constant relationship with various systems of self-representation.

More precisely, he states that various systems of self-representation are active within the ambit of every social group, and that these interact among themselves, and with the language of daily life, developing a function of reflection, and more generally of production of sense. Lotman examines in particular the part played by the theatre, literature, painting, the cinema and fashion. His research shows that:

- The theatre and the other forms of artistic expression mentioned above give a representation (at various levels) of social reality.

- The representation may even have as yet unformed sketches of behaviour and feelings in an embryonic state as its object.

- The activity of representing them, of acting upon them, promotes their formalisation.

- This also means that such behaviour and feelings reach a higher degree of expressiveness and communicability.

In Lotman's model the function of self-representation is not expressed by a single film or dramatic work, but by the whole production of a certain period. Nevertheless, an example is useful, even if it refers to a single work. Between the end of the 1950s and the beginning of the 1960s, in the petty bourgeoisie and also among the 'common people' of Rome there was a widespread, naive and optimistic desire to 'be American'. The film *Un Americano a Roma,* thanks to Alberto Sordi's ironic and highly emotional interpretation, painted a vivid picture of these collective feelings and hopes. By providing an enjoyable and well-defined image of this home-spun form of 'Americanism', the film also contributed to getting over the behaviour it depicted.

Work of representation

A new representation in a small analytic group may at first be denied, to reappear in another form, after further thought. It may be refuted yet again, reappear again, and finally be accepted. A self-representation which relates in an authentic and dynamic way to what is evolving within the group causes friction. It is hard for the group members to accept this self-representation because it implies accepting being different from what they had thought themselves to be up to that moment.

One of Melanie Klein's ideas is useful when considering the work of representation. She states that what attracts the love (and the destructiveness) of the small baby is the internal part of its mother's body. The internal part of its mother's body is seen by the baby as the very fountain of creativity, and appears rich in precious and fascinating things to its eyes. I believe that in phantasy there is a superimposition of the internal part of the mother's body on the internal part of the group, and the representation of the group coincides with exploring and becoming aware of what exists in these obscure and productive spaces.

The dream as language

Returning to Lotman's model, I should like to point out that the systems of self-representation – in his model the theatre, literature and cinema – are in the small group essentially built up of dreams, phantasies and imaginative speculation. These are not the only systems of self-representation active in the small group. For example, certain types of behaviour occurring in the group may also have a self-representational function. However, the three systems of self-representation I have mentioned (dream, phantasy and imaginative speculation) are a particularly good 'fabric' for expressing desires, agitations and what is not known and causes conflict.

I shall now speak in particular of one of the three systems of self-representation indicated, i.e. the dream. Considering the dream as a system of self-representation means seeing it not only as a 'product' which can be interpreted, but also as a true representation of 'something' which the person has picked up and worked through (in an unconscious and preconscious way). More precisely, it is the expression, representation and working through of what is happening in his internal world as well as in the analytic situation in which he is involved.

This way of understanding the dream is not all that far from Freud's, except for one point which is, however, fairly substantial. I am referring to the idea that the content of the dream undergoes considerable deformation and masking due to censorship.

The dream as a newspaper

Freud considers the analysis of dreams as an instrument which makes it possible to reach the desires of early infancy which have been repressed, and precisely because of this have remained immune from the passing of time. However, the road through to the unconscious is not easy; in fact it requires interpretive work and a determined emotive working through. In fact, the desires present in the dream are hidden and protected by the work which censorship has done on them to prevent them arousing a reaction of the inner judgmental authority (Super-ego). In Freud's opinion (1900) 'The dream is like a newspaper in a dictatorial regime which absolutely must come out every day, but must never tell the truth, and the work of the editors is to cover up the truth as much as possible or tell it between the lines' (see Mancia 1993, p.9).

Meltzer (1984) suggests that the dream be considered, not as a deformed expression, but rather as a true expression of unconscious desires and phantasies, but one which is expressed through a language different from the verbal one.

More precisely, Meltzer's idea is to extend the concept of language by including the dream in it, considering it as an inner language or rather as a poetic or creative language which describes the inner world. His idea clarifies what I am referring to when I speak of the dream as a system of self-representation.

A WC-bus

A clinical example may be helpful here.

> One of the participants (Massimo) brought this dream to the second session of a therapeutic group: 'I was at my group, but it was also a bus or perhaps a big four-wheel drive … There were other people there but I couldn't make them out very well … I was sitting in the driver's seat.
>
> Something was happening … after this event I became aware of a smell … Then I realised that I was not sitting on a seat, but on a WC. Each seat was a WC.'

I want to linger over this dream and suggest an interpretation. The following interpretation, however, is not the one given in the session, but more of a study intended to bring out points which are relevant to the theme being treated.

As I have already said several times, I do not think the leader's role consists so much of interpreting as of keeping spaces open for working through, and of enabling the group to move to and fro between reason and emotion, between living out a fear situation and preventing fear from becoming panic.

My observations relating more directly to the patient (Massimo) who told the dream can be summed up as follows:

- In the course of the group's first session, the patient, as he himself declared when associating on his dream, had been extremely anxious and tense and had been afraid of losing emotional control (the group was…a big four-wheel drive).
- To protect himself from the possibility of being emotionally overwhelmed, he dreams of taking the part of the analyst and himself driving/leading the bus/group (he was in the driver's seat). This attitude – as I shall understand better in the successive course of the analysis – reveals a specific aspect of the structure of his character.
- Something happens (probably 'what happens' is one of my interventions in the course of the session). After this, the patient is able to draw attention to his own emotional state ('he became aware of a smell').
- The awareness of his own emotional state permits him to realise that he is not the only one to feel the effects of being in the group (each seat is a WC).

The contributions of the dream to self-representation of the group are:

- The indication of the confusion which pervades the group (there were other people there, but I couldn't make them out very well).
- The individuation of a common tendency to get rid of emotions – and particularly fear – without letting them be seen (wetting oneself).

- The image of a first collective 'container' (the bus).

Personal dreams and dreams for the group

The dream I have reported offers contributions both to the representation of the dreamer's state of mind (fear of losing control, taking the driver's seat) and the representation of the group (indication of the confusion and fear which reign in the group, image of the group as a bus). All the dreams that are told in the course of a group analysis contribute in two ways, individual and group. However, a few points need specifying. The fact that a person brings a dream to a group does not imply that the dream becomes a group dream, even if it is the group which receives it and works it through. This assimilation would imply the negation of the contemporaneous presence of both individual and group dimensions in every dream (not to mention in each of the members' interventions) and would constitute a really undue appropriation by the group.

Moreover, it is necessary to distinguish between various types of dream. Some dreams communicate above all something which is proper to the individual, as though the dreamer were making a gift of a fragment of his own childhood, or a precious photograph from his family album, to the group and to the analyst.

In these dreams the group is the recipient of the dream, rather than what is represented in the dream. In other dreams the story of the individual is in the background, and in the foreground there is an image of the group which may be represented through the persons who are a part of it, or through a phantasy personage who condenses the whole group into a single figure (for example, the figure of a rapist) or through a symbol (for example, the light of a candle). In yet other cases, the dream is a message for the group. It is something which is essential to the group's existence and is communicated through a dream.

A historical example is Joseph's dream told in the Bible, in which the seven fat cows and the seven lean cows warn the Egyptians to reflect on their condition and their future.

When a dream is made for the group the dreamer often prefaces the telling with a phrase such as 'I believe that what I dreamed relates to the situation which has been created here.' Giving this presentation he shows that he is aware of having carried out a 'duty' for the group. He has kept his ears open and become receptive to the deep moods of the group; he has worked through these moods and synthesised them in the images of his dream. When the task is finished, he wants the analyst and the other members to appreciate this.

Self-image and group representation

The members' self-representations go step by step with the group representations that are gradually produced. Ernesto's dream, reported below, illustrates this point. The session in which the dream was told took place about two years after the beginning of treatment.

> We had organised ourselves in groups of five or six to explore an underground city.

> I had brought with me a large amount of luggage but had discarded some of it, because several people had advised me to do so in view of the difficulty of the journey. So, before starting, I had opened my pack and left in it just the essentials: an electric torch, a bottle of water, two or three ready-made sandwiches and a bar of chocolate. We were in single file and I was at the back. At a certain point we found ourselves in a big open space where there were lots of people of different races and ages: children, old people, individuals of all kinds. I felt really terrified because I did not know who these people were, what they were doing or what they wanted. The others could no longer be seen. I also began to feel physical pain: cold, and a need to be sick.

> I began to retreat, little by little, into a tunnel. Then I felt someone touching me. It was my maternal grandmother, who had looked after me when I was small. My grandmother said to me: 'How hungry and cold you are. I shall have to do something for you.' She then moved back to a place where the tunnel opened out into a little space. She sat down and began to prepare food. It was primitive food: beans and coarse bread.

> I was still very anxious, but I was beginning to tell myself I ought to look for the others.

> My grandmother said: 'But if you don't eat and get warm, you won't even be able to look for the others.' I sat down, too, and looking at the ground, in the light of the fire which my grandmother had lit in order to cook, I saw something. I realised it was the shadows of the others who were coming near. (I should like to thank Dr. Fortunata Gatti who led the group analysis session during which this dream was told.)

In the dream, Ernesto turns to his grandmother, who has had a maternal function, and to the group after being lost in the big open space of the underground cave. In reality Ernesto had recently become aware that he had become isolated from the other members, and more generally from others in his life.

Therefore, his return is also an escape from isolation. In the dream of the underground journey, this awareness of his own isolation is shown by the fact that Ernesto sees himself at the end of the queue. In another dream of the same period Ernesto is in a room and suddenly realises that there is a pane of glass or crystal between himself and the other members of the group. Encouraged by someone present, he pushes against this pane with all his strength. At a certain point, he is conscious of great pain, and then the glass gives way.

However, on returning to the group, Ernesto did not go back to the position he had previously been in. The dreamer after being lost and no longer being able to recognise his surroundings, having felt lonely and desperate, returns with an awareness of his personal needs, which are also essential needs.

The representation of the group, given in the dream, is also progressively modified. At the beginning it is the image of a few people giving advice on the luggage to be taken. Then it transforms into a multitude in which he is lost. At the end of the journey it has become the 'inner image' of a group of people coming near, seen through the reflection of the fire on which his grandmother is preparing food.

A multi-dimensional whole

This is the right moment to provide a more detailed notion of semiosphere of which I gave an initial definition in the introduction to this chapter. The semiosphere corresponds, at a semiotic level, to the unity of the group and to the creation of a common sensorial and emotive area, that is, the group's common space. It also corresponds, at a representational level, to what the field is at a depository level and at a level of creating a system of interdependence.

The term semiosphere indicates more precisely the ensemble of systems of self-representation and of other systems of sense-determination which operate within the group, and also indicates the semeiotic continuum within which these systems operate.

As I have already mentioned, in the small group the self-representation systems are above all dreams, phantasies and imaginative speculation. The general discourse of the group, because of the analytical setting, also becomes an expression of collective states of mind which are not directly observable and which can be very different (and sometimes in opposition) to those expressed verbally by the members of the group.

Technique

The concept of self-representation offers the analyst the possibility of referring, not to a predetermined idea of the group, but to an idea which is gradually presented in the self-representations offered by the participants. This results in a group image subject to successive transformations in which emotions and phantasies are particularly relevant.

The concept of semiosphere allows the therapist to calibrate some dimensions of his interpretive function in an optimal way. The notion of semiosphere, in fact, allows interpretation to be seen as a system of self-representation and production of sense, which works alongside others and finds its own specificity, not when it superimposes on other systems, but when it keeps their work going. I am referring once again to the dream. In the dream there is working through and interpretation which, so to speak, belongs to the dream itself. The therapist – who takes into account the idea of semiosphere – with his interpretation places himself within the group associative chain (of which the telling of the dream is a link) and creates the conditions for the continuation of the dream-work (see Wittgenstein 1919).

PART 4

Group Thought

The part of this book dealing with group thought represents a development of themes which I began to outline in the last chapter of the preceding section on the semiosphere. I shall also take up again some points discussed in the first chapter, regarding the group associative chain and the star-shaped arrangement. In the first chapter of this part of the book, 'Brain and Mind', I shall tackle the following themes:

- somatic and sensorial basis of thought
- super-individual thought units
- thought of individuals and group thought.

The two brief following chapters, 'Characteristics of Group Thought' and 'Therapeutic Function of Group Thought' aim at explaining how:

- the thought of individuals and the thought of the group can enter into a relationship of natural collaboration.

Finally, in the last two chapters I will consider the conditions necessary for the development of group thought with a psychoanalytic function. In particular, attention will be drawn to:

- the relationship between unexpressed and expressed (mimesis)
- oscillations between emotions and thought.

CHAPTER 8

Brain and Mind

Freud in *The Interpretation of Dreams* (1900) defines the psychic apparatus by comparing it to optical instruments. The arguments he develops make it possible to assert that in his theory the psychic apparatus is not understood in the anatomical sense. More generally, it can be said that for Freud the psychic apparatus is taken as a model, or, as he claimed himself, has the value of a fiction (see Laplanche and Pontalis 1967).

Bion (1970) establishes a closer link between brain and mind. He maintains in fact that the apparatus for thinking thoughts is the result of a kind of functional restructuring of the brain. More precisely, according to Bion, the brain was originally made for various tasks, and only later – under the pressure of new necessities – did it adapt to house thoughts.

Bion's idea can be clarified by a few words of illustration. An individual faced with a dead person, a corpse, may deny the sense of this image: for example, he may think that it is a hallucination. A group faced with an unexpected happening (a stone falling) may move instantly and flee like a flock of birds. Thus, fear is not a thought or an experience, but something from which one escapes directly by recourse to hallucination or flight (see Cupelloni 1983).

We should add that taking on the burden of thinking thoughts and not getting rid of them in the form of action but keeping them within the mind as representations, as scenery, creates anxiety, both because of the content and because it implies a detachment from man as a group animal. The individual who, seeing the falling stone or the corpse, does not flee with the rest, feels persecuted not only by what he thinks, but also by the fact that he is the only one to be detached from what everyone else sees as a 'vital' or 'life-loving' reaction. By taking on the burden of thought, the individual becomes a lone animal and is therefore threatened by reason of his very isolation from the herd. It is here that we can locate the passing from the brain as the protobrain to the brain as a mind, the container and elaborator of thought (see Agosta 1988, pp.227–236).

Primitive thought and evolved thought

I shall complete my treatment of Bion's theory of thought with a few more notes. Bion does not make the usual distinction between cognitive and affective. He considers thought in a way identical with emotion. For Bion, and for psychoanalysis in general, thought is also intensely cathected by emotions when it is taken into the mind as food, as something which makes it grow. The second characteristic of Bion's way of describing thoughts consists of differentiating between 'technological thought' and 'thought which takes the responsibility of thought'. This distinction has already been partly suggested by those French authors who speak of 'operative thought'. Bion, however, develops the theme in a different way. The transformation of the 'protobrain' into mind does not, according to Bion, imply the acquisition of greater technological ability. It is not a question of being able to carry out increasingly sophisticated conceptual, algebraic, mathematical and logical operations, but of being able to take on the responsibility of the images, scenarios, effects and contents of thought. From Bion's point of view, thought capable of designing the atomic bomb is not necessarily more evolved than that of monkeys fleeing or attacking *en masse*. It is technologically more advanced but has not necessarily interiorised the responsibility of thinking of violence, aggression and death.

The third characteristic of thought highlighted by Bion corresponds to the capacity of thoughts to promote the development of the mind. The mind, which hosts thoughts (what the eyes see, intuitions, things that happen), does not get rid of them, but keeps them, gives them a form, links them with emotions, dresses them in words which make it possible to communicate them, expands, evolves, and becomes more and more able to live through experiences. An incapacity for thought, on the contrary, is a diminishing of the human being and corresponds to a large extent to the contemporaneous or successive appearance of various manifestations of a psychiatric type. I shall illustrate these ideas with some images taken from a film by S. Kubrick.

> The film *2001, a Space Odyssey* begins with a herd of monkeys behaving savagely. Then unexpectedly a monolith or stele appears, the meaning of which the monkeys are unable to understand. They begin to move more and more agitatedly around this object. One of the apes takes a long bone and begins to use it to break other animals' bones and skulls.

> While he is playing in this way, he suddenly becomes serious, as though struck by an intuition.

> In the following scene, the apes are drinking from a pool.

> A horde of rival apes appears, which up to then has always forced them to retreat. The ape which had picked up the bone and found out how to use it stands up to them and kills some of them.

Then the scene takes a great leap into the space age. A space ship is starting out on an exploration. The appearance of the stele is the reference point of a significant new evolution.

A computer within the space ship which is heading for Jupiter, the computer called Al begins to become conscious of itself

This computer is highly developed from the point of view of capacity for technological thought, but is still quite incapable of bearing frustration. At a certain point it miscalculates the temporal resistance of a part of the space ship and is contradicted by another computer on earth. Al cannot bear the frustration and in a terrible rage kills the astronauts.

In the first scenes of this film we see the moment in which thought capable of discovering instruments appears; a bone can be used as a hammer. This discovery, however, is immediately subject to the primitive impulse of 'attack or flee'. The images of the space ship represent a very advanced stage of the technological evolution of thought. The computer Al is in fact an example of highly developed technological thought which nevertheless remains tied and subjected to an inability to articulate feelings which give a sense to oneself and one's limits.

I shall add two more very short notes. The first is that according to Bion the possibility of taking on responsibility for thought involves two stages: one of distancing oneself from the group (acceptance of one's own solitude) which is followed by fresh acceptance of belonging to the group. The second is the realisation that we do not cross the threshold of thought as a responsibility once and for all, capacity for thought must be constantly reacquired.

Co-existence of primitive thought and evolved thought

We have seen how the mind and capacity responsible for thought are an evolution of the primitive brain (protobrain). However, according to Bion, the primitive brain continues to be active, even when a mind that works with evolved thought has developed. This hypothesis corresponds to McLean's theory (1970) on the existence in man's brain of three brains (reptilian, of early mammals, of modern mammals).

Reptilian brain and brain of early and modern mammals

In the course of evolution, the brain of primates has developed according to three main models, which can be qualified as the reptilian model, the model of early or primitive mammals and the model of the later or evolved mammal. The result is an interesting mixture of three cerebral types which differ radically in their chemical mechanisms and structure, and which are independent in an evolutionary sense. There exists, so to speak, a hierarchy which unites the three brains into one; this is what I have called the one-and-three brain. Although the three brains are closely interconnected and functionally depend on each other, it has been shown that each is capable of operating independently of the other two.

The reptile brain includes the reticular and striate forms. It is the seat of individual and species survival. The behaviour it generates is automatic and invariable; it offers no possibility of adjustment to changes in the environment. The second brain, that of early mammals, corresponds to the limbic system. It is the seat of motivations and emotions; it is capable of responding to present information by appealing to the memory of past information. The third brain is represented by the neocortex. In particular virtue of its frontal position, it is the brain of anticipation, capable of choosing the response to a stimulus as a function of the effect it will have, based on the memory of effects it has met in the past. It is the most evolved brain, that of 'intelligence', characteristic of the higher vertebrates; this gives individuals a high degree of adaptability and therefore greater liberty. (Vincent 1986, pp.124–126)

I should like to submit that there is also in the group something which, in correspondence with McLean's model, could be called the 'collective primitive brain' which co-exists with a 'collective evolved brain' or group mind.

For this hypothesis to be consistent I must first explain what I mean by group brain. Neurones or nerve fibres do not pass between persons forming a group, but there are methods of communication based on hormones which operate at a distance (pherormones). For example, in all species of vertebrates, and also in man, it has been found that steroid hormones govern various types of psychosexual behaviour. There are also mental and sensorial channels based on numerous patterns such as muscular tension, bodily position, the rhythm of breathing. Electroencephalographic research carried out by Hobson, Spagna and Earls (1977) on married couples who share the same bed and show synchronisation of REM and non-REM sleep patterns are also indicative in this sense.

When speaking of the 'collective primitive brain' I shall be referring globally to those communication channels which are largely automatic and unconscious (see Lindauer 1990, p.156; Massa 1979, p.225).

Studies by E.N. Marais (1921, pp.72 and 45) on termite colonies may help to envisage how a 'collective primitive brain' functions:

The Eutermes termites build huge anthills more than five metres high, within which the humidity remains the same throughout the year. These ant-hills have wells more than fifty metres deep with a complex arched architectural structure. Marais' observations on this type of termite can be summarised in four points:

1. All the movements of the individual termite are governed from outside, by signals which regulate the entire functioning of the ant-hill. The termite as an individual has not the slightest trace of free will nor power of choice. The only quality the termite possesses is self-mobility, the ability to move. It starts to move of its own accord, but when a given movement has to be made, the aim of this movement is established and directed from outside. Circumstances may render the termite's work useless; this happens for example when there is an obstacle in its way that it can neither confront nor avoid; in these cases in which the simplest individually controlled insect would try to escape, the termite does not stop.

2. There is an influence, a thread which firmly binds the termites together. This influence works through various types of communication (sonar, hormonal, biochemical) and also through a community signal. The community signal serves to hold the community together and allows each termite to recognise every other member of the community.

3. Distance lessens the influence. It works only within certain fixed limits.

4. The death of the queen immediately cancels out any influence. Damage and wounds weaken this influence in proportion to the extent of the damage.

W.R. Bion described something similar to the ant-hill when he spoke of the basic level of a group's mental life: a level at which people operate by responding to collective stimuli with automatic replies. At this basic level the behaviour of the members (and of the group as a whole) is directed by a rudimentary collective brain: the protomental system.

I am convinced that Bion's view on the basic levels of thought (protomental system, primitive mentality, basic assumptions) points to some important aspects of group function at a basic level such as automatism, impulsiveness, inability to reflect, a trans-individual character. I believe however that Bion's protomental model does not throw sufficient light on another equally important aspect of the primitive mental life of the group. I mean the connection between the basic levels (sensorial, somatic, emotive, preverbal) of the functioning of the group mind and the more evolved aspects which operate at a symbolic level.

The protomental system

According to Bion (1961, p.111 sqq.) we cannot understand the sphere of protomental events if we refer solely to the individual; it is in groups of individuals that we find territory suited to an understanding of the dynamics of protomental phenomena. The protomental stage in the individual is only part of the protomental system.

In the protomental sphere the individual is part of a system, even when a distinction has been made at other mental levels. The image of a mushroombed may help. Observing a mushroom-bed one sees the individual fungi separated from each other and scattered over a large area of ground but an infrared photograph would show not the fungi, but the network joining them. The 'network' of the protomental system is not directly visible but if it is damaged, the damage appears in the suffering or ailing of one or more of the elements (the fungi scattered over the ground).

Phenomena at the protomental state are both somatic and psychic at the same time. Bion represents the protomental system as something in which the physical and the psychological or mental are not differentiated. These protomental levels form the matrix of illnesses (for example tuberculosis) which appear in the individual, but have characteristics which show that it is the group that is affected.

It is also from the protomental system that all-comprising collective phantasies, defined by Bion as basic assumptions, emerge.

The basic level functioning of the group may be positive or negative, but in either case it has many connections with the levels of sentiments, passions and thoughts. These connections vary according to events; but certainly they are not as automatic and uninfluenced as the idea of basic assumptions and the protomental system would lead us to believe. At certain moments the experience of someone leading a small analytic group may appear to confirm Bion's view; at other times, however, it is not so. It is difficult to realise when the basic dimension in the group is more of a wide physical, sensorial and affective dimension, capable of providing affective containment and support, and when on the contrary it is something which is obsolete, automatic and non-evolutionary. It is even more difficult to understand what the factors are which make group functioning incline towards one or the other of the two dimensions. Something may be said with regard to functions of the type I described in Chapter 5 as the Genius loci of the group, that is to say, functions which take account of the group's syncretic identity.

Superior type super-individual thinking units

The basic level of relationships proper to the protomental stage and syncretic sociality is not the only one operating in the group mind, which also functions at very high levels of complexity and differentiation. At a higher level we can properly speak of the relationship between many and one, between individual minds and the group mind. McDougall (1927, p.9), who is interested in this evolved level of group functioning, considers the 'group mind' as a particular group and relational reality. According to his definition, the group mind is an organised system of mental forces; a system which is no part of the mind of any individual, but is, rather, made up of the relationships which exist between the minds of the individuals who constitute it.

The existence of a culture and the presence of a group language are factors which distinguish the primitive level of group function from the evolved level. I have already dealt with this theme, though in different terms, in Chapter 6, when illustrating the notion of the 'historical field of the group'; I shall now add only a few short observations. J. Goodall (1990, p.229) notes: 'Sometimes, observing chimpanzees, I have had the feeling that not having a human-type language they are in a certain sense prisoners of themselves.' Goodall's phrase reflects something I have often felt when taking part in group sessions. There are moments, fairly rare in reality, when we get the impression that language is bringing us out of isolation, giving us not only sensorial and emotive participation in the group, but also thought contact, contact between minds. These moments are probably the optimum moments of the functioning of the group as a superior super-individual thinking unit.

On the subject of language I should also like to stress that a small analytic group develops its own language. Chomsky's studies (1977) show the ability of small groups to create their own language; they show how the dialects of gangs of youths in New York or Los Angeles are understood as actual languages and not as sub-products of, or deviations from, a hypothetical 'standard English'. Naturally the languages of small youth groups are based on the English generally spoken in their community, but they have their own autonomy, are closely linked up with the history and culture of that group, and have a vitality of their own. As languages they serve to express basic contents for that group. They also represent a characteristic which distinguishes each group from the others.

Making space

Another characteristic which distinguishes the group mind (as an elevated super-individual unit) from the basic levels of the 'primitive collective brain' (comparable to the anthill) is that every single individuality which becomes a part of it is still a whole with specific characteristics. In the anthill, the ants doing their various tasks (as workers, warriors, queen etc.) specialise and lose their initial potentiality. In the 'group mind' working at an elevated level, the individual does not lose his capacity for individual thought. (see Corrao 1981, p.26; 1982, p.23; Tinbergen 1953, pp.179–85).

Numerous consequences derive from the co-existence of individual thought and group thought, a co-existence which characterises the functioning of the group mind as a super-individual unit at a high level. One of these is that at this high level of the 'group mind' there is no automatic or compulsory communication between the group and the individuals as happens at lower levels. It is necessary for communication to be sought and constantly adjusted.

If the group mind (as an entity working at a high level) and the individual mind are to enter into a relationship, both the group and individuals must have reached a certain degree of evolution. As far as the group is concerned, this happens at the Fraternal Community stage. This collective subject, the Fraternal Community, is the carrier of group thought and becomes the interlocutor of the individual members. From the individual point of view, taking part in group thought at an evolved level requires the capacity to be available as a link and work through other people's thoughts. This is not always an easy operation. In fact, it means receiving 'thoughts which are circulating' without feeling invaded, annulled or unduly influenced by them. Becoming available for other people's thoughts also implies being able to make space within oneself, to make time for waiting which is not only experienced as emptiness and anxiety. With regard to this, a very different situation from that of the group comes to mind – a love relationship. A girl complained to her grandmother that the refrigerator was always full for a lover who never came to see her. The old lady suggested: Try emptying it, then you will see that he will come. In terms of group analysis: making space becomes possible when one's own affective existence does not depend too directly on confirmation and recognition by the analyst and the other members. It is therefore easier if the analyst and the other members first try to understand and respect the point of view of the person who is going to be asked to make room for the others (see Di Leone 1993; Marinelli 1993)

Syntony

Another condition necessary for communication between individual thought and group thought is the establishment of syntony. The individual feels that the thought of the group – at least partly – is autonomous and independent of him; if there is no syntony, he feels that it is inaccessible rather than autonomous. If syntony is established, he feels that it is something he can confront, and to which it is worth contributing. D. Stern has used the term attunement to indicate the process which leads to the establishment of syntony between a newborn baby and its mother, and the consequent passage of communication. Attunement is regulating which can preserve individual characteristics and at the same time promote functioning as a whole. Each individual can maintain his own way of thinking which is characteristic of his phase of development, and at the same time take part in the functioning of the whole. More specifically, Stern's idea is that affective intensity, rhythm and time provide a 'transmodal interface' able to link up different thought structures, without cancelling out their differences. When I speak of syntony between individual thought and group thought, I am referring to something of this sort.

Attunement

The process of attunement in the mother-baby dyad is as follows: the mother gathers the baby's signals (gurgling, way of crying, movements etc.) and reproduces them transmodally. The term 'transmodally' makes clear how a sensorial modality, for example the sounds of the newborn (gurgling, crying), is reproduced in its mother's motor-sensorial register. The baby sees a toy, and in trying to get to it says 'Aaaah'. The mother watches it, and watched in her turn, stretches her body (motor-sensorial register) with an intensity, time and rhythm analogous to the baby's 'Aaaah' (sound and auditory register).

Similarly a baby's movement may be transformed into a sound uttered by its mother. In this way a dialogue is established between the mother and her baby (see Imbasciati 1991, p.127; Stern 1985).

CHAPTER 9

Characteristics of Group Thought

People are often dubious about what is produced by group thought. In Latin the saying is: *Senatori boni viri, senatus male bestia*, which means that senators as individuals, taken one at a time, are good people, but taken all together they degenerate. And yet there is a completely opposite traditional Russian theory: the *mujik*, the peasant, is considered stupid, but the *mujiki* council, formed by the heads of peasant families, is deemed intelligent.

Both opinions, whatever we may think of them, maintain one essential point, that the characteristics acquired by the group as an entity capable of thought are not equivalent to the sum of individual qualities. On the contrary, these characteristics depend on a series of factors which determine the characteristics of the collective as a thinking entity.

Thought of the small analytic group

I shall now limit my discourse to the thought of the analytic group.

The people taking part in a group analysis are present in the same room, therefore, group thought in the analytic situation corresponds to the experience of 'thinking together'.

Moreover, in the small analytic group, the setting is particularly important in the development of discourse, which is very different to that found in ordinary social situations outside the analytic setting.

I am referring, in particular, to the setting up of the analytic chain which I dealt with in Chapter 1. At certain times, in the small group, the discourse 'free-wheels' when a certain word sparks off a thought, and that thought a word (anacrusis), and the total result is a rich articulation of images, emotions and ideas. Another aspect of communication proper to the small group which I should like to mention is the 'star formation'. When the group functions in this way, the development of the discussion proceeds spontaneously with the confrontation of different points of view on the same subject (syncrisis) and with the superimposition of images (thematic amplification). This results in bringing to light a meaning which is present, but implicit and which would not otherwise be very evident.

The small analytic group also works with an alternance of verbal thought and images. An example is given in the telling of dreams, which, no matter how different their contents, acts like an enzyme which can cause an acceleration in the communication and the work of the group, by transporting the categories of the discourse into a visual space.

This means that thought, in the small analytic group, is extremely mobile and varied and has many facets (see Lotman 1993, p.52; Perelman and Olbrechts-Tyteca 1958).

Globality and versatility

In the analytic situation, thought works on various elements (thoughts, emotions, phantasies) which correspond to a common 'field'. Consequently transformation concerns at the same time all the interdependent elements, so that when one is modified, the whole is modified. A picture of the globality of the transformation with which group thought operates is given by the game of 'Cat's Cradle'.

The game of 'Cat's Cradle' is played with a piece of string about 50 cm long, with the ends tied together.

By weaving the string between the fingers of the two hands, the first pattern is formed.

The player who intervenes (normally it is a game for two, but there may be more than two players) takes the same piece of string from the first player and, according to the way in which he does this, modifies the pattern which has been passed to him.

S.H. Foulkes has suggested a phenomenon which considers another aspect of the globality of group thought, i.e. polarisation. Polarisation in optics corresponds to the phenomenon of the rainbow, and also of the small rainbows produced by white light when it passes through a prism. As we know, white light is the result of the sum of a series of emissions of various wavelengths. Passing through a prism the ray is divided according to the different wavelengths making the various colours in the white light visible. In the same way, according to Foulkes (1964, p.317) in an analytic group an emotional and phantasy nucleus is subdivided into the elements that constitute it. Each of these is taken up and represented by different individuals. The total reaction of the group as a whole is the result of the sum or combination of these partial responses. A clinical account gives an illustration of polarisation in a small analytic group.

> At the beginning of the session, one of the patients participating in a group which has met weekly for a year says that this time she has been feeling anxious about coming to the group.

Several other members phantasise about why she is feeling anxious. One of them says that he is expecting the women to speak in this session. Another tells of a complementary phantasy: when he arrived there were only women there, and he thought the women had got rid of all the men. At this point a lively debate develops on the theme: is sexuality compulsory in the group?

A young woman intervenes strongly, affirming that the tendency to live as though sexuality were a necessity does not make sense. Several examples are given, including the one of Rosy Bindi, a Christian Democrat parliamentarian, who supports the value of virginity.

The analyst says that sexuality is certainly not compulsory, but if there is sexual tension in the group it is difficult not to feel its effects. The woman who started the discussion says she was feeling anxious because she is pregnant.

'I would have started my sexual life earlier, or had a more straightforward sexual life, if I had not been anxious about getting pregnant.'

The question opened up and various people spoke about wanted and unwanted children.

This illustration shows how a series of phantasies projected by various members of the group (how they waited for the women to express themselves, the idea of the elimination of the men, their anxiety about sexuality) are the effects of the dividing up of a strongly anxiogenic and 'very unreal' nucleus concerning pregnancy and the possibility of becoming pregnant through participation in the group.

CHAPTER 10

Therapeutic Function
of Group Thought

Metabolic capacity

One of the primary aspects of the therapeutic function of group thought is its capacity to metabolise anxiety and anguish, which the individual may not be able to work through on his own. In other words, the group has the capacity to free the individual's mind from excessive tensions which may have accumulated. To express this idea in a different way, it might be said that group thought has a function analogous to that of an individual's alpha function.

Bion gives us a picture of how the α-function operates. It is commonly said that if a person has a nightmare, then it is caused by indigestion – somatic indigestion. However, we could also imagine the nightmare to be the result of mental indigestion. During the course of the day, an individual accumulates a series of experiences and is involved in emotional situations which he is unable to metabolise. The effect of this accumulation is a nightmare. In fact, Bion distinguishes a nightmare from a dream. He says a nightmare has an evacuatory and hallucinatory quality. The anxiety accompanying it is the sign that the psychic apparatus has been overwhelmed and has not managed to digest certain experiences. On the contrary, a dream is the result of the alpha function's work, that is to say, the transformation operated by the alpha function on the emotional experiences which have accumulated.

The therapeutic function of group thought – as I was saying – appears first of all as the capacity for working through anxiety. Every one of us has sometimes felt exhausted and depressed at night, and felt incapable of thinking. If we are in a warm environment, in a convivial group situation, this helps to make us feel better, even if the activity taking place in the group meeting is in itself intense and exhausting. Francesco Corrao (1981) calls this metabolic function of group thought, γ-function (group function). γ-function is analogous to α-function. The use of the Greek letter γ corresponds to the idea that what activates this function is not an individual, but a group. The γ-function is, when all is said and done, the capacity of group thought to 'metabolise' sensorial elements, tensions and fragments of emotion which are present in the field.

A thought which operates outside the individual

Carrao's hypothesis, that group thought has a metabolic capacity, can be usefully linked with some of Searles' hypotheses.

However, before referring to Searles' hypotheses, it might be a good idea to spend a few words on putting his studies into context. Basically, Searles deals with two themes, the treatment of very serious patients and the problem of the relationship between the individual and the environment, where environment is both human and non-human.

With reference to psychiatric departments of hospitals and the teams who work there, Searles has stated that treatment for serious patients requires certain mental functions to be initially activated outside the individual (in the team) and that only later can the individual come into possession of them. This is the point I should like to 'connect up' to the metabolic capacity of group thought. Searles says: (1965, pp.315–317):

> The clearest and simplest way of describing the type of social situation which the patient with the fragmented ego tends to create in the department is, in my opinion, to consider this social situation as a process through which the distinction and later integration of the different fragments of the ego must take place to a great extent outside the patient himself, in the persons surrounding him, before they can happen within him.

The 'seriously ill patient' who succeeds in using the team to activate those mental processes which he lacks, probably lives his life as one with the team. The phantasy of fusion with the team enables him to take advantage of its working through activity, without feeling he has anything to do with any object different from himself.

The team is in fact a part of his mind.

I believe that the process described by Searles is true not only in the hospital team, but also in small analytic groups, and that not only seriously ill patients can benefit from it, but all patients taking part in group analysis.

A space for thought

Another aspect of the therapeutic relationship established between the individual and the group is that group thought may offer a sort of spatial support to the thoughts of the individual. In other words, I am referring to the fact that the individual may take the versatile structure of the group as a 'special space' offered to his thoughts. In this case there is no necessity for a phantasy of fusion with the group, as the individual's thought proceeds alongside that of the group. This is what a patient who was particularly capable of introspection, said to me in the course of a conversation following the end of his group analysis:

> Sometimes in the course of a session a problem came to my mind which at that moment I could not or did not wish to tell the other members and the analyst. The choice of not speaking about it could arise from the fact that the group discussion in that phase was very active and emotionally intense, and I did not want to introduce a new theme. On other occasions it was a decision founded on the fact that I did not feel quite ready to communicate my very confused feelings.

> Therefore, on such occasions, rather than force myself to talk about what was worrying me, I preferred to follow attentively the other members' discussion. Not that I tried to remove the problem from my mind. It was ever more present in my mind as the group discussion went on.

> At a certain point I saw a connection between a detail of the theme which was being discussed in the group and my problem, as though a bridge were being built between my thoughts and what was said in the group. The intersection of my thoughts and the thought of the group then allowed me to find an original approach to the problem which was worrying me. That is to say, it became possible for me to consider the problem from a particular angle, as though I had taken my place in a new and significant emotional scenario. I found solutions which I had not thought about.

Another patient noted how essential it was for him that the group analysis had offered him 'space for listening'. This patient once said: 'Only a few times, when I spoke in the group, did I receive a reply, but more than in any other place, what I said was listened to.'

Psychoanalysis has sometimes spoken of the 'sensitive mother'. This 'sensitivity' is also innate in the analytic group, in the sense that even the tiniest word is listened to. Paradoxically, at certain times the members of the group may seem distant or uninterested regarding the individual who is intervening and his problems. This is not insensitivity, but rather a way of distancing themselves from arguments which are difficult to face in a group, in order to have time to think about them and then come to a definite conclusion. I am constantly surprised at how the members of a group remember all the details of what a person has said, which seemed to have passed unobserved months earlier (see Boccanegra 1994, p.1).

Technique

I shall conclude the chapter with a final short observation on technique. In the analytic group, discussion need not necessarily lead to a unitary synthesis. On the contrary, various points of view may be taken into account at the same time. This makes it easier for the participants, through a multi-faceted identification with the different viewpoints present in the group, to be delighted at meeting up with some characteristic which is also a part of their thought.

CHAPTER II

Conditions for Group Thought

The presence of the group

What conditions are necessary for group thought to be able to operate effectively in a small analytic group?

Perhaps the most important condition is that there should be what I shall call the 'presence of the group'. Clearly it is essential that the people in the group should be physically and mentally present. But what I mean is that a point of reference should be created, that a certain quality of emotions should be condensed and a phantasy relating to the existence of the group should be formed. The 'presence of the group' is in fact a phantasy, but also a 'fictional reality' (but still a reality) which people refer to when they introduce a discourse. The 'presence of the group' is one of the elements which gives depth and frequency to group thought, because the members all realise when speaking that they are not only referring to one another, but also to another common point.

To make the argument more effective, I shall use some passages from *To the Lighthouse* (1927) by Virginia Woolf.

> The situation in *To the Lighthouse* is one of a group of people, the Ramsay family together with their friends and acquaintances, who meet in a country house. Against this background the idea of a boat trip to the lighthouse takes shape. One particularly significant moment is a dinner party organised by Mrs Ramsay. At the beginning there are no ties, the guests are all seated separately.

> 'Lily was listening; Mrs. Ramsay was listening; they were all listening. Lily felt that something was lacking; Mr Bankes felt that something was lacking ... Mrs. Ramsay felt that something was lacking. All of them bending themselves to listen thought: ... "The others are feeling this ... Whereas, I feel nothing at all".' This is the zero moment, the moment of departure in which the presence of the group is not yet there; people have gathered together but they are all on their own, there are no ties. Several people, including Lily and Bankes, feel uncomfortable, but one person in particular realises that it is up to her to make an effort to remedy the awkward situation. Mrs. Ramsay thinks that 'the whole of the ef-

fort of merging and flowing and creating rested on her. She felt, as a fact … if she did not do it nobody would do it'.

'She turned to Mr Bankes who was isolated from the others and feeling awkward.

"How you must detest dining in this bear garden," she said, making use, as she did when she was distracted, of her social manner. So, when there is a strife of tongues at some meeting, the chairman, to obtain unity, suggests that everyone shall speak in French. Perhaps it is bad French; French may not contain the words that express the speaker's thoughts; nevertheless speaking French imposes some order, some uniformity. Replying to her in the same language, Mr Bankes said, "No, not at all".'

Virginia Woolf says that Mrs Ramsay speaks distractedly, in a worldly style, but that her intervention is effective. A first trace of what is to become 'the presence of the group' appears. A conventional language is proposed, but it is a common one.

Mrs Ramsay keeps up the effort of 'merging, flowing and creating', even establishing emotive agreements: 'things' may be seen in very different ways by different people yet despite this there can be co-participation. At a certain point of the dinner a dish of fruit appears on the table.

'Thus brought suddenly into the light, it seemed possessed of great size and depth, was like a world in which one could take one's staff and climb up hills, she thought, or go down into valleys, and to her pleasure (for it brought them into sympathy momentarily) she saw that Augustus too feasted his eyes on the same plate of fruit, plunged in, broke off a bloom there, a tassel here, and returned, after feasting, to his hive. That was his way of looking, different from hers. But looking together united them.'

Virginia Woolf describes two very different ways of approaching a common object, a big dish of fruit. Mrs. Ramsay's way is being able to walk through the dish of fruit as she were walking through the mountains while Augustus's is that of a bee furtively gathering a little pollen. But his eyes and Mrs Ramsay's meet over the same dish. A non-verbal language creates sympathy and convergence. This is a second feature which contributes to the creation of group presence.

The transformation, which Mrs. Ramsay had been preparing for a long time, happens almost by magic.

'Now all the candles were lit, and the faces on both sides of the table were brought nearer by the candle light and composed, as they had not been in the twilight, into a party round a table, for the night was now shut off by panes of glass, which, far from giving any accurate view of the outside world, rippled it so strangely that here, inside the room, seemed to be order and dry land; there, outside, a reflection in which things wavered and vanished, waterily.'

Suddenly, it is as if the windows no longer permit a view of the outside, but reflect back the images of the inside. The inside is cosy, and becomes attractive to the members of the group. The outside loses interest. They are all concentrating on the situation. At this point, Mrs. Ramsay's guests are no longer what they had been in the twilight. At this point the 'presence of the group' has been created, i.e. a common situation, a feeling of being there, of being gathered together.

Presence of the group and common space

In Virginia Woolf's story, the sensation of the presence of the group is accompanied by the perception of the existence of the group's common space. Both these phenomena coincide with the arrival on the table of a dish which it had taken three days to prepare – a beef casserole in red wine with herbs and onions. The arrival of this dish offers an emotionally-loaded object to be shared.

> 'Here, she [Mrs Ramsay] felt ... was the still space that lies about the heart of things, where one could move stay or rest; could wait now ... listening, could then ... sink on laughter easily, resting her whole weight upon what at the other end of the table her husband was saying.'

Mrs Ramsay – now, like each of the guests – could let herself go with her thoughts and phantasies. And they would find a welcome.

She lets this 'admirable fabric' of thoughts and words support her and sustain her, so she can totally abandon herself to it. 'Then she woke up. It was still being fabricated.'

A constellation

Now we shall leave aside Mrs Ramsay's dinner for a moment, to turn to the conditions which are necessary for effective functioning of group thought. If these conditions are to be fulfilled, besides the 'group presence' there must be also the presence of a 'constellation of phantasies, emotions, feelings, thoughts'. If group thought is to operate effectively it is not sufficient to simply speak of dependence or admiration or melancholy, but dependence or admiration or melancholy and the procession of phantasies which accompanies each of these feelings must be actually present in the field. (see Hautmann 1985).

Why a constellation? From the thousands of stars in the sky, we sometimes single out eight or ten stars and imagine them to be joined up. When we join them together forming the constellation of the Plough or the constellation of the Pleiades, they acquire significance.

These stars stand out from all the others and become recognisable. I believe that something similar happens in the group.

Before Mrs. Ramsay's dinner party begins, there is dispersion, the feelings which animate the guests are changeable and not clearly defined. Then an emotive-phantasmatic constellation appears which is centred around the phantasy of a liaison between Mrs Ramsay's son and a house guest, a girl called Minta.

Now we can take up the thread of the story again. Mrs. Ramsay wonders where the two have gone to. She is worried. When she is told that they have come back, she discovers a feeling which she had not expected. She had believed she would be relieved by their return, and instead she feels angry.

"'They've come back!" she exclaimed, and at once she felt much more annoyed with them than relieved. Then she wondered, had it happened? She would go down and they would tell her – but no. They could not tell her anything, with all these people about. So she must go down and begin dinner and wait.'

Waiting pervades the whole group gathered for dinner. The conversation of the guests includes sentences which seem to indicate that even if the constellation is still indistinct, it is nevertheless already active. Above all, there is curiosity, associated with some rather bizarre phantasies.

"'It's odd that one scarcely gets anything worth having by post, yet one always wants one's letters." Said Mr Bankes ... "Do you write many letters, Mr Tansley?" asked Mrs. Ramsay ... Had Carrie written to him herself? "Yes. She says they're building a new billiard room," he said. No! no! That was out of the question! Building a billiard room? It seemed to her impossible.'

Virginia Woolf is notably ironic about the phantasies relating to the engagement. It is compared to the idea of the construction of a billiard room.

At a certain point, having to remain in suspense, without a reply, causes annoyance. But then something happens.

"'I lost my brooch – my grandmother's brooch" said Minta with a sound of lamentation in her voice and a suffusion in her large brown eyes, looking down ... It must have happened then, thought Mrs. Ramsay, they are engaged. And for a moment she felt what she had never expected to feel again – jealousy. For he, her husband, felt it too – Minta's glow ...

"'When did Minta lose her brooch?"

'He smiled the most exquisite smile, veiled by memory, tinged by dreams.'

Mrs Ramsay is partly right and partly wrong to be jealous. She is right in that another woman seems to be taking her place, establishing a special relationship with her men, but she is wrong because her husband, in Minta, is remembering her, finding her once more and passing the baton to the following generation. In asking about Minta's brooch, Mrs Ramsey's husband is passing on something precious to the new generation [Minta and Paul]. He is implicitly evoking a moment, many years before, when she too [Mrs Ramsay] had 'lost her grandmother's brooch' with him [Mr Ramsay]. The brief question 'When did Minta lose her brooch?' contains an intense and deep-felt idea of temporality. Here we see an example of how each of the members of the group can experience the same emotive-phantasmatic constellation (the engagement) at the same time yet each with his own references, calling up memories which he can only partially express or not express at all to the other participants.

The conversation of Mrs Ramsay's guests then turns to other themes, however many of them seem to be somehow aware that something has happened. Mrs Ramsay is certainly aware.

'"Ah, but how long do you think it'll last?" said somebody. It was as if she had antennae trembling out from her, which, intercepting certain sentences, forced them upon her attention. This was one of them ... "Let us enjoy what we do enjoy," he [William Bankes] said. His integrity seemed to Mrs. Ramsay quite admirable ... She liked Charles Tansley, she thought, suddenly. She liked his laugh. She liked him for being so angry with Paul and Minta.'

The dinner is over.

'It was necessary now to carry everything a step further ... she moved and took Minta's arm and left the room.'

CHAPTER 12

Mimesis

I should like to examine in greater detail the relationship established between the phantasmatic constellation, which I began talking about in the preceding chapter, and the level of group discussion.

However, even before beginning this examination, I should like to explain that when I use the expression 'level of the discussion' I am referring both to what is explicit and what is hidden, even if it is not possible to identify it at first. In fact, group discussion may also communicate other than what is immediately apparent.

In the course of Mrs Ramsay's dinner, which was the main thread of the last chapter, the members of the group speak about a billiard table, whether they get letters or not, and of a brooch that has been lost. These discussions, apart from their obvious meaning, also establish a relationship with something which is not explicit, but which nevertheless gives them particular intensity.

Mimesis

The nature of the relationship which is established between the elements of the discussion and those of the 'emotive-phantasmatic constellation' active in the group can be explained by applying an idea of W. Benjamin (1933) regarding mimetic ability. The notion of mimesis (or 'mimetic imitation') in Plato's philosophy indicates the imitative relationship which links ideas with what is tangible. Ideas are to a certain degree prototypes and they appear in the world of tangible things through a process of mimesis, or imitation. It should be emphasised that the terms mimesis and imitation – both in common speech and in Plato's works – suggest a passive and gregarious repetition and a certain impoverishment with respect to the original, since an imitation is a copy. However, Aristotle differs from Plato in giving a positive value to mimesis, emphasising its cognitive value.

Benjamin goes further, saying that the relationship established through mimesis is an active relationship and that it is not simply a cognitive operation. The relationship created between the 'tangible image' which imitates, and the idea, or 'intensifying constellation', cannot be described by saying simply that the first is a representation of the second (the constellation); mimesis means at one and the same time representing something and 'making it present' in the very situation in which the representation occurs.

Transformation in K and evolution in O

In order to clarify this aspect of the mimetic function we may usefully turn to the distinction established by Bion between evolution in O and transformation in K.

Transformation in K indicates Knowledge, that is, being informed about something. While in using the terms evolution or transformation in O Bion is referring to becoming something.

If we apply Bion's concept to the idea that in the group there is an emotive-phantasmatic constellation on which mimesis operates, we can hypothesise that the speaking activity in certain circumstances may have the capacity to stimulate the constellation to specify itself, to evolve towards the field of the known. At the same time group discourse can be influenced by the presence of this constellation, so that this same discourse would receive particular constellation contact characteristics. Instead of speaking of a constellation, we might use the term pool, that is, a collection of sensations, emotions, and still unformed phantasies which may be present in the background of the group field, and are then gradually defined. Or we may speak of 'O', of an evolutionary element in transformation which influences the very life of the group. On this subject, A. Correale (1991, p.245) makes the following notes:

> The analytic group is sometimes pervaded by an emotion which cannot find adequate definition in the expressive capacity of the group itself [then thanks to the fact that it has entered into contact with an evolutionary nucleus, and to the construction of a system of transformations, the emotion which could not be represented beforehand] slowly acquires consistency and transmittability.

Evolution in 'O'

For Bion, growth is an effect of thought which knows (K) but above all of the evolution of reality itself (evolution in 'O'). The first form of transformation (K) can be described as a thought analogous to knowing about something, that is, it responds to the clarifying function of analysis. However, amplification of knowledge of this type (K) cannot be the only function of analysis. When we are dealing with the reality of personality, something more than an exhortation to 'know yourself' and 'accept yourself' comes into play. The point under discussion is how to pass from knowing about phenomena to being what is real. In analysis, the process responsible for the development of new mental facts has been defined by Bion as 'evolution in O'.

Evolution in O does not mean knowing phantasies or other already evolved forms of mental activity, but getting into unison with what is not yet evolved and stimulating it to grow and differentiate. This development (evolution in O) necessarily implies the activation of tensions, which are related to forces and terrors which only religion has dealt with up to now. Interpretations which being about the transition from 'knowing about' psychic reality to 'becoming' psychic reality (transformation in O) are feared and create resistance. However, for Bion this transition from K to O (from knowing to becoming O) is fundamental for the growth of the mind (see Grinberg et al. 1972, p.130).

Effectiveness of mimesis

Returning to mimesis, it can be asserted that it is through mimesis that tension between 'O' and the level of group communication is built up.

Benjamin reminds us that in antiquity it was believed that it was the mimetic faculty which permitted the establishment of a relationship between a given community and cosmic forces. For example, the construction of a temple began when the relationship between the celestial constellation which was beginning to appear and what was being initiated promised to release favourable energies into the enterprise. It was thought, in fact, that there was a mimetic relationship between the favourable forces of the emerging state of the cosmos (the rising constellation) and the emerging state of the other object (the beginning of the construction of the temple) and that favourable cosmic energy could be transmitted to the microcosmos.

Benjamin also mentions that in antiquity it was believed that mimetic relationship could be activated through appropriate ceremonies. There might be a dance which imitated the movement of the cosmos, and through this dance a contact could be established between the microcosmos (the community) and the macrocosmos (the movement of the stars). The extraordinary dance of the 'whirling dervishes' which imitates cosmic movement is not only a representation of the cosmos, but it is an actualisation of cosmic forces. The whirling dervishes are a mystic Islamic sect which originated with the great poet Rumi who came to Konia from southern Anatolia. The dervishes begin their dance by spinning round and round. The dancers as an ensemble also spin around until they reach a state of collective mystic intoxication. This dance reactivates the relationship between the cosmos and the dervish community.

The group in its activity of thoughts and words operates a mimetic relationship with what is neither said nor expressed, with a constellation which is still being formed and defined. And gradually in the course of the session the group picks out, chooses and gives form to something.

On other occasions, what is 'actualised' through mimetic imitation is not a constellation or an emotion of the group, but a deep-down experience of one of the participants.

On this subject, it should be noted that the correspondence established through mimesis does not imply that the participant's experience is reproduced by the group with the same themes used by that individual. On the contrary, the points of correspondence may be 'immaterial resemblances'. For example, the group may note the presence of an extremely significant state of mind in one of its members which, nevertheless, remains unexpressed because he cannot put into words what he is experiencing. What may happen then is that the group ignores the individual's theme, but represents its negative, its opposite, or presents it in an extremely transformed way.

The individual will still note that the group's discourse has an essential, deep relationship with his state of mind (see Gaburri 1992).

Concreteness of mimesis in the group

W. Benjamin (1933, p.71) speaks about immaterial resemblances when describing a playing child. While playing and imitating, a child can capture a movement, the strength of the wind or the quality of a person: 'The child does not only play at being a shopkeeper or a teacher, but also at being a windmill or a train.'

Mimesis, carried out by the playing child, is not only representation. The child chooses a particular element (strength, movement) of an external figure (e.g. a windmill). A feeling comes to life (admiration, awe). The related choice and feeling is accompanied by identification with the object. The child becomes the object and at the same time assumes its 'quality'.

At Mrs Ramsay's dinner, treated at length in the last chapter, when the constellation centred around the engagement phantasy is specified, a tasty dish on which particular care has been lavished (stew in red wine) arrives on the table.

Sharing the engagement-related emotions and phantasies corresponds to the sharing of the *boeuf en daube*. Here is a last passage of *To the Lighthouse* in which the

interweaving of the engagement phantasies and the appearance of the main dish
of the dinner is particularly evident.

> '"We went back to look for Minta's brooch." He [Paul] said, sitting down by her.
> "We" – that was enough. She [Mrs Ramsey] knew from the effort, the rise in his
> voice to surmount a difficult word that it was the first time he had said "we".
> "We" did this, "We" did that. They'll say that all their lives, she thought, and an
> exquisite scent of olives and oil and juice rose from the great brown dish ... and
> she [Mrs Ramsey] must take great care. Mrs Ramsay thought, diving into the
> soft mass to choose a specially tender piece for William Bankes. And she peered
> into the dish, with its shining walls and its confusion of savoury brown and yel-
> low meats, and its bay leaves and its wine, and thought, this will celebrate the
> occasion – a curious sense rising in her, at once freakish and tender, of celebrat-
> ing a festival, as if two emotions were called up in her, one profound – for what
> could be more serious than the love of a man for a woman, what more com-
> manding, more impressive, bearing in its bosom the seeds of death; And at the
> same time, these lovers, these people entering into illusion glittering eyed, must
> be danced around with mockery, decorated with garlands.'

Mrs Ramsay compares the idea of the consummation of a marriage to the image
and the sensations of a spoon sinking into the dish of beef with onion. In the
small analytic group sharing means sitting together. It implies going through
phantasies which are seen in a very concrete way, and even as hallucinations.
Mimesis in the group corresponds to the activation of more primitive functions
than those envisaged in the image of the playing child. The experience can be
very concrete and lively. While the child's game might be thought of as a phantasy activity, in the case of the group, if something is imitated and captured
through mimesis there is an almost hallucinatory presence. The coupling of
Minta and Paul – in Mrs Ramsay's thought – becomes white and dark meat into
which the spoon or the knife is plunged; or else the pot becomes the womb
which contains the force of germinative seeds and of death. The child plays at
being the windmill and becomes the force of the mill. The group actually sees
and eats the *boeuf en daube*. The child gathers the force of the mill; the members
of the group gather the essence of mating and eat it in the *boeuf en daube*. In a
small group they not only speak about the sea, but also bathe in it.

Despite this concreteness, using mimesis to make something 'real' – in the small
group – does not exclude, but is rather accompanied by, a later distancing process in order to obtain knowing and transforming. There is an immediate making of contact, but following that there is the possibility of knowing (see Barnà
1993; Bonazza 1993; Pomar 1994).

Technique

I am going to make one last observation on the role of the group analyst. The analyst's empathic process in a group is different from the one he activates in the

traditional psychoanalytic situation. In the latter the analyst accepts an emotional state of the other person. On the other hand, in the group, the analyst, through empathy (or perhaps, more precisely, through an emotional intuition) accepts not so much the atmosphere of the session, but the constellation behind it. In this way he facilitates the realisation of the group's mimetic processes, and can also make it possible for the other group members to get into unison with 'O'.

CHAPTER 13

Oscillations between Passions and Thought

I shall conclude the section of the book devoted to group thought by dealing synthetically with the theme of the relationship between knowledge and emotional participation.

The classical concept and the psychoanalytical concept

According to classical philosophic tradition – initiated by the Stoics, by Epicurus and by Seneca – passion and knowledge are in opposition. Passions subject men to fluctuations of the mind, stopping them from obtaining adequate knowledge of what they are experiencing while exposing them to unending conflict. According to this tradition, knowledge may be compared to a ray of light falling on a basin full of water; the more movement there is in the water in the basin, the more the possibility of seeing anything clearly is lost. Even if the ray of light is well directed and falls in a straight line, vision is distorted (see Bodei 1991, p.315). The psychoanalytic method diverges from classical doctrine and develops a different approach to knowledge.

Psychoanalysis regards the passions as a form of knowledge. Consequently, it is not centred around the problem of the clash between passion and knowledge, but, rather, concentrates on the conditions which allow a passionate, participating observer to reach into knowledge.

What is more, psychoanalysis does not separate knowledge from the process that the subject who knows has to face. Rather, it maintains that the person undergoes a substantial transformation during the cognitive process which he himself has started by taking part in the analytic situation.

From the point of view of psychoanalysis, knowledge is not an exchange of intellectual possibilities, but corresponds to the development of the capacity to transform profoundly.

Finally, psychoanalysis does not consider repression of passions a desirable or in any way pursuable aim. Nor is the transformation which is sought through analytic therapy reached by a deadening of the emotions, or through a well-amalgamated mixture of passions of an opposite sort. The psychoanalytic paradigm is the metamorphosis of passions into emotions. In other words, passions, knowledge and relationships are thrown into dynamic collation. The bond thus created will promote greater stability in the person and make it possible for him to derive satisfaction from reaching the goals that, every now and then, knowledge and passion will be able to reach (see Bodei 1991, p.283).

Oscillations

The method of approach which I have outlined is to be seen in technical instructions regarding the analyst's assumption of a specific mental attitude. Freud speaks of fluctuating attention or correctly distributed attention. Bion of actively renouncing memory, desire and the search for reasoned explanations. The analyst in addition must eschew any form of moralistic or abstract judgement. Lastly, it is indispensable that he should always try to bring to light any possible complementary aspects of passions and thought. This mental attitude on the part of the analyst, in its turn, favours a particular type of group functioning. In fact, in every session there will be oscillations between moments of emotive and passionate participation, and moments of reflection which are the premise to an integration of passions and thought (see Corrao 1992, pp.15–16; Falci 1990, pp.74–83).

Destructuring

Continuous spontaneous transformations of thought and passions can sometimes lead to a block. If this happens the entire functioning of the group can be greatly hindered and even impeded. The impossibility of experiencing and knowing about a certain feeling (for example, depression and sense of loss) can take the form of a mental state (for example, a sense of oppression) which pervades the majority of the members and appears as soon as the group meets. On other occasions the cessation of oscillation between passions and thought is a consequence of the fact that there has been a process of institutionalisation of beliefs, emotions and phantasies, which have become empty and stereotyped ceremonies. On yet other occasions the difficulty may take the form of division of the group into two opposing sub-groups, which put obstacles in each other's way and cause reciprocal stabilisation. In these circumstances Bion speaks of a 'schism'.

In certain cases the analyst has to encourage the bond in order to cope with these block situations. At other times he has to make sure that the best security conditions for the bond are determined. For example, security allows interventions by those members of the group who can and wish to present very intimate thoughts and emotions. Their silence may depend on the fact that the group condition is so intensely fiery and passionate that they prefer to remain in the calmer and protected position of being silent observers. If the analyst introduces quieter tones, these members feel 'authorised' to express what they have in their minds. The complex work of the group regains efficacy thanks to their contribution (see Baruzzi 1980).

On yet other occasions it is not a matter of encouraging the creation of greater security conditions, but rather of destructuring a defensive and paralysing 'affective-cognitive aggregate' which is operating in a hidden way, blocking the group. The operation of destructuring can take various forms. For example, the active and sudden one of a 'happening' or 'brain-storming', or the gradual and continuous one of work with associations and interpretations, or the subtle and specific one of the perception of a question, hidden and waiting beyond (or in the middle of) the block or the turbulence. In all cases, the objective of destructuring is the dismantling of ideology, verbal constructions and defensive strategies, in order to allow thoughts to take their place in emerging emotional contexts (or 'emotive fields'). This also makes it easy for the individual members of the group to abandon their islands of 'non-participation' which may be protecting them but at the same time are preventing them from contributing to and benefiting from the thought of the group. (see Bodei 1994; Corrao 1985, p.15).

Destructuring is a painful moment because a pre-existant mental attitude is put in a critical position. And even if this pre-existant attitude was full of discomfort, it was still, in a certain sense, known and considered protective. To explain this more clearly, I shall illustrate these assertions with a story which belongs to the tradition of a branch of Buddhism.

> The spiritual head of a community of Buddhist monks has died. A general assembly is taking place with a dual purpose: to choose the future spiritual head and to define afresh the essence of Buddha (Buddhism, the founding thought of the community).
>
> Many of the monks are speaking in a knowledgeable way. Those present, however, remain uncertain and static. Things are difficult. Thoughts are not making contact with feelings. The community is prevented from making fresh contact with the vital founding centre, with 'O'.
>
> One monk stands up. His attitude and aspect are modest. He is the community's cook. He is holding a cooking pot, but then he opens his hands and lets the pot fall to the ground. The cooking pot breaks into a thousand pieces. Those present perceive their loss in a concrete way. The pot is a container, like the old spiritual head. However, the essential thing about a pot, or a container is the emptiness it contains. A pot is useful because it is empty inside.
>
> Those present realise that they can make contact with their feelings (the breaking, the loss, the confusion) again and with the thought which constitutes the

real value and the nourishment of the community: emptiness, Buddha, the un-saturated.

The destructuring of a pre-existing group attitude always implies feelings of loss and confusion. But if loss and confusion are tolerated long enough – with a con-tinuing associative and thinking activity – a new direction and a new sense can emerge in the group.

PART 5

Group and Individual

This section of the book is divided into different chapters:

- Chapter 14: On new members joining the group
- Chapter 15: The group's reaction to the entry of new members

Themes which have already been examined in other parts of the volume, (self-representation of the group and representation of self, Emerging state of the group), are taken up again and considered from the specific angle of the relationship between group and individual.

The following chapter of this section:

- Chapter 16: The group as self-object

goes more deeply into the study of the group as an object of affective cathexis, which I touched on briefly when speaking of the Fraternal Community stage, and in particular when I introduced the notion of the group's affective heritage.

The last two chapters:

- Chapter 17: Effective narration
- Chapter 18: Transtemporal diffusion

complete the part dealing with the notions of the group's common space, the Field and the Semiosphere, considering the relationship between the Field and the experiences of the individuals who are taking part in the group.

CHAPTER 14

On New Members Joining the Group

In the first part of the book I described the way in which participants, going through the phase of the Emerging state of the group, converge towards common mental states. The description was based on clinical material from small groups formed by individuals who had all begun analysis together. However, another possibility is that of a 'semi-open group', where periodically some members leave the group, having completed their analytic work, and new participants join the already-formed group which is continuing to function.

In this chapter I should like to consider a semi-open group and the entry of two new members (Luigi and Marzia). When they enter the group, Luigi and Marzia form images, which allow us to follow closely the development of a relationship between individuals and the group. In particular, we will be able to see how the new members imagine both the other individuals and the group as having a skin, and how becoming members of the group is seen by the two new participants as really 'getting inside' the group.

Encasings

I shall come straight to the point, presenting the first significant contributions of the two new members. They are a phantasy of Luigi's and a dream of Marzia's, which are brought into the third session after their arrival.

> (*Luigi*)

> 'I was thinking that if we were able to run faster than the speed of light, we would little by little meet up with our past. But now I realise that if we slowed down, even for a moment, the spaceship in which we were travelling would crash into us.'

Luigi had imagined analysis as a very fast mental journey into the past, but he found himself facing a spaceship-group which risked colliding with him if he interrupted his giddy speed of thought by allowing himself a single pause.

(*Marzia*)

'I dreamt about a tortoise with a baby tortoise on its back. The big one was constantly struggling and I thought perhaps it couldn't tolerate the little one.

At a certain point the little one fell off and lay upside down with its feet in the air. I looked at it and saw on its side a little patch of mould, as though it were ill. The big tortoise meanwhile continued to be agitated, so I realised that its restlessness was not caused by the little tortoise.

I thought that if the little tortoise were ill, the big one might be as well, so I turned it upside down and on its stomach there was a mouldy patch like a peach gets when it has been lying on one side for a long time. I should have liked to touch it with my finger to see if the shell was still hard, but I was afraid my finger would sink in.

Marzia compares the group and herself to two tortoises. She dreams of being balanced on the surface of the group (the little tortoise is precariously balanced on top of the big one).

She perceives a great restlessness in the group (the big tortoise struggles constantly) and wonders whether she is the cause of this restlessness (she thought that the big tortoise could not tolerate the little one).

The little tortoise is pushed away (the little one fell). This allows the dreamer to verify that the group's restlessness is independent of the presence of the little tortoise. In addition, the fall makes it possible to see the underside of the tortoise (it lay upside-down). It is a female tortoise and perhaps this coincides with being ill (it had a little patch of mould on its side).

The big tortoise is also like the little one. Marzia tries to penetrate inside it, but is afraid of losing herself (it was a mouldy patch ... she would have liked to touch it with her finger ... but she was afraid it might sink in).

CHAPTER 15

The Group's Reaction to the Entry of New Members

Before presenting the clinical material which will serve as illustration to the chapter, I should like to emphasise that a member who comes into an already formed group (even if it was formed only a few sessions before) is seen by the other participants (the founding members) as a person who joins an already defined and perfected whole. On the contrary, if that person had been present from the beginning, he would have been considered as part of the original Gestalt. The entry of a new member, after this Gestalt has been fixed, involves a complex restructuring of the group as a whole.

An initiation rite

I shall present the same sequences considered in the preceding chapter, but seen from the point of view of the new members.

At first the original members do not seem at all interested in the new arrivals (Luigi and Marzia). This probably depends on the fact that their arrival coincides with a fresh start of sessions after the summer holidays, and the 'old' members are too busy repossessing the group to bother about them. This dream, told in the course of the first session after the summer holiday, is indicative of phantasies related to taking possession of the group again:

(*Marzia*)

I took various volumes of the *Brain Research* collection from the shelves of the library where I work.

The volumes changed into chairs, and I went round and round sitting on each of them.

Gradually the stomach cramps from which I had been suffering all summer diminished, and finally disappeared.

However, I was frightened by a voice from off-stage. The voice said that the moves I had already made did not count and I would have to start again from the beginning.

In Marzia's dream, just as in an initial rite, one after another there is: the reanimation of memories (I took volumes from the *Brain Research* archives); the identification of Marzia with each of the members (I sat on each of the chairs); the depositing in the group of anxiety experienced during the summer (going round and round ... my stomach cramps disappeared). However, in the background (off-stage) we can see anxiety over the annulment of the efforts previously made (the moves already made did not count).

Group and anti-group

In the following sessions the old members began to notice the presence of Marzia and Luigi. Some dreams and phantasies, which I am not reporting, show that the old members do not consider Marzia and Luigi as two people, but as members (or parts) of another group (an anti-group) which is trying to break through the group's boundaries, but without deciding to really do so.

There is expectation, hope, and a climate of almost unreal suspense. Even the feelings of hostility aroused by the arrival of the new members are suspended in an almost motionless aura. These feelings, as I was saying, are not directed at them as individuals, but at their role as representatives (or messengers) of a hypothetical other group which is approaching. The presence of analogous feelings has been effectively expressed by C.P. Cavafy (1908) in his poem 'Waiting for the Barbarians':

> What are we waiting for, assembled in the forum?
> The barbarians are due here today.
> Why isn't anything going on in the Senate?
> Why are the senators sitting there without legislating?
> Because the barbarians are coming today.
> What is the point of senators making laws now?
> Once the barbarians are here they will do the legislating.

The old members: the returning dead

After a few sessions, the waiting takes on a more definite form. A phantasy appears that the new members are 'the returning dead'. The expression 'returning dead' refers to a few members of the original group who had abandoned it for various reasons, leaving a series of negative feelings. This association of Pietro (in the sixth session) marks the most organised and also the most violent expression of the phantasy of invasion by the living dead.

(*Pietro*)

I read that researchers in various parts of the world, working on tissue cultures, got a glimpse of particular phenomena. This raised hopes of a good result.

It was then seen that the phenomena observed were HeLa cells. They are cells of a black woman who had died of cancer in 1955, HeLa cells, so called after Henriette Lax.

These cells had been extracted from the cerebral, or rather cerebellar tumour of which the woman had died. Various laboratories chose them because they reproduce with great rapidity and remain unchanged for successive generations.

Now they are appearing in other tissue cultures where they had not been expected and where they had not been cultivated.

A researcher is collecting data on how many laboratories are polluted.

Pietro is expressing anxiety that what he had sought to keep away was present in the group (the cells of Henriette Lax appeared in cultures where their presence was not foreseen).

However, he also seems to recognise that the appearance of these cells (the appearance of new members) is a product of group research (various laboratories had chosen and isolated these cells). We can perhaps hypothesise that the HeLa cells are the incarnation of the primitive part of the group mind which is appearing in its field-laboratory.

Observations

In following sessions in which Pietro relates the history of the HeLa cells, a comprehensive reconstruction of the group starts which will allow the full participation of Marzia and Luigi. I shall not however linger over these developments, instead I want to propose some observations of a general nature.

In fact, the clinical material seems to me sufficient to advance a few hypotheses which complete the subject proposed in Chapter 2, concerning the creation of a group boundary.

- The distinction between old and new members corresponds to the distinction between the inside and the outside of the group. The entry of new members breaks through the boundary which marks this distinction.

- The group is trying to transform the unknown into something which is already present in its code (the anti-group, the returning dead).

- The entry of one or more new members is never simply an assimilation. If a new member is really to enter and take part, the group must undergo a comprehensive restructuring. The destructurisation and restructurisation of the group implies the re-emergence of phenomena of the Emerging state of the group (expectation, hope, persecutory anxiety, depersonalisation).

CHAPTER 16

The Group as Self-object

In this chapter I shall take up once more points relating to the group's affective heritage, which I have already dealt with in Chapter 3 – in the Fraternal Community stage. I shall also treat some aspects of the argument regarding the therapeutic potential of the group which I have not yet tackled.

Some therapeutic functions of the group

When there is an adequate development in the analysis, the group gives the participants an experience of belonging, something which is very important for the construction (or reconstruction) of the sense of Self as a person who has the right to exist and occupy an affective space. For many patients this right has not been adequately recognised in their family environment during childhood. The group provides them with an important experience of belonging and of affirmation of their right to exist. The paradoxical condition of 'being here without existing' has been effectively expressed by Buñuel in *Le Fantome de la Liberté,* a film about a little girl who lives in her family but is never seen or heard. For her mother and father she does not exist.

The group also gives the participants the possibility of improving their own self-esteem. The improvement in self-esteem is closely linked to the progress of the group. In fact, the importance which the members attribute to good collective functioning depends not only on the need to maintain the illusory idea of the group as a sort of Paradise (group illusion). Another fundamental reason is that the reconstruction of their self-esteem is linked, to a considerable extent, to the success of a collective undertaking to bring into existence a worthwhile and capable group. Third, being in the group gives the participants the sense of an opening up of possibilities which helps them even in everyday activities. In a training group, one of the participants, for a joke, put a poster on a wall of the room in which the sessions took place. It showed an advertisement for a small fork-lift

truck, and underneath the name of the firm which produced it was written the slo-
gan: 'The force of a large group to take the weight off your shoulders.'

The capacity of the group to develop these therapeutic functions, and in particular its ability to be of support to the people taking part in it, depends to a large
extent on the integrity of all those elements which have been cathected with the
participants' emotions and which, as we have seen, constitute a sort of affective
heritage of the group.

Among these elements are: the fact that the group is 'complete' (or almost);
that there is continuity of sessions; the absence of events which could disturb stability; a constant emotive and material environment. On the contrary, any
disturbance that concerns the structure of the group (for example, the arrival of
one or more new members) puts at risk the possibility that participants can use it
to gain strength and security and deal with their own internal and external difficulties (see Correale 1991, p.78; Kohut 1984).

Another effect that the group has in establishing a positive relationship with
those taking part in it may be indicated by the word 'animation'. As a result of a
positive relationship with the group, certain aspects of the patients' personalities,
which have always been present but hitherto have been silent and unexpressed,
come to life and acquire depth and intensity. After leaving Friuli and moving to
the suburbs of Rome, Pasolini (1957) wrote some lines which illustrate the emotional state to which I am referring:

> I was in the centre of the world, in that world
> of sad Bedouin districts
> of yellow meadows slashed
> by a relentless wind.
> Whether it comes from the hot sea of Fiumicino,
> or from the countryside, where the town was lost
> among the hovels.
> A soul within me, which was not only mine,
> a little soul, in that unbounded world,
> grew, fed by joy.

The group as Self-object

In the situations which I mentioned in the first pages of this chapter, the relationship of the individual with the group is not one in which there is a subject with a
distinct object which is cathected with desire, but one in which the relationship is
with something which is only partially differentiated.

As far as individual analysis is concerned, this perspective has been developed
by H. Kohut who speaks of Self-object relationships. According to Kohut, the
Self-object is neither Self nor the object, but the subjective aspect of a support
function of Self, activated by the relationship which Self establishes with those

objects which through their presence and activity bring out and maintain Self and the experience of being themselves. So, the object-Self is a function of the subject indissolubly tied up with the presence of a real object (see Wolf 1988).

There are various types of Self-object relationships. Each type is characterised by a particular function:

- twin or alter-ego Self-object
- ideal Self-object
- mirror Self-object.

The basic idea of the twin Self-object relates to a reflection on the terrifying possibility, experienced in a more or less accentuated form by everyone once or twice in a lifetime, of feeling that one 'is not a human being' but a monster or a robot. Contrary to what one might think, the fact of being a 'human being' is not a certainty acquired with birth, it has to be confirmed by others. In other words, everyone needs someone else to present and confirm his 'being human' for him. We could lengthen the argument by speaking of the need for a human environment that can guarantee 'being human'. The twin Self-object (or alter-ego Self-object) provides a continual presence, which is not only intellectual, but also physical; this presence makes an essential contribution to the construction of the feeling of being 'human among humans'.

We are talking about the experience of taking part and being safe, because of the assured presence of other people (voices, odours, emotions, sounds etc.). Anyone who has children or remembers the time when he was a child, knows that paradoxically children sleep better, not when there is absolute silence, but when they hear people talking and moving about, maybe in the next room. Family sounds accompany the child at the moment when, on falling asleep, he loses his points of reference.

Hearing human noises assures him of the presence of his context, of not being transported into a world in which he could, like the child in the story of the Wizard of Oz, become a tin man.

The synchronisation of the breathing of people together in one room, the propagation of anxiety, the simultaneous activation of menstrual cycles in a number of women, correspond to experiences which can be related to the twin object-Self, and which, in a previous chapter, I examined with reference to J. Bleger's concept of syncretic sociality. The experience of relationship with a twin object-Self is much more marked in group than in individual analyses, because the physical presence of other people (the analyst and the other members) is more consistent and explicit. In the group, more than in the dual analytic situation, the sight of people, physical contact, movements and the presence of an active and functioning assent, are of great importance. On this subject G. Trentini (1987, p.45) writes: 'The group represents for the individual an important source of confidence and certainty…capable of satisfying any subjective anxiety about this basic need which is present in every individual.' This capacity of the group is particularly important for those patients who are suffering because their feelings of existing and being themselves are not well structured.

The central idea contained in the concept of ideal Self-object is that the perfection of the primitive omnipotent Self is transferred to an object. This object is idealised but not distanced. The ideal Self-object is seen more as an extension of Self. Consequently, the experience which comes from a relationship with an ideal Self-object is that of being at one with 'an ideal of calm and strength' (see Pallier 1992).

The process of omnipotence transference described by H. Kohut, which is not accompanied by a separation or distancing of the object to which the omnipotence has been transferred, is significantly different from the one that Freud and Bion regard as optimal. According to Bion, it is essential that the moment of birth of the ego ideal and the transfer of omnipotence and omniscience to this ideal (i.e. to an entity 'external' to the subject) should be accompanied by discrimination between itself as bounded and the ideal object. Kohut's notion of the relationship with the ideal Self-object, on the other hand, maintains the importance that this transfer should not bring about an inevitable detachment between the subject and the object which is holding ideality. If this detachment is too traumatic and radical, the subject remains emptied and impoverished. If, on the other hand, a phantasy of non-distinction is maintained, the subject can continue to have access to ideality (to omnipotence and omniscience) which is located in a person (the 'grown-up', the father) who is really capable. This 'grown-up', however, is seen as being available for the child and in a certain sense controllable by him. The image is one of a child on his parent's shoulders. For example, for one patient of mine having an Alsatian dog was extremely important. This young woman had transferred to the dog the strength, power, courage and defensive ability that she could not exert. Through the dog, she felt safe even when she was alone in the house because the dog could protect her.

Relationship with the ideal Self-object is the basis of a certain anti-depressant effect of group therapy. The group is a giant compared to the individual. Consequently, the group as an ideal Self-object, puts at the participants' disposal a certain amount of 'omnipotence which can be shared and utilised'.

Besides the experience of sharing omnipotence, the ideal Self-object can mirror a joyful reflection of the conquests achieved by the subject, giving him a positive image. This experience is comparable to being in a ray of light, as if there were a spotlight following and shedding light on one. This makes it possible to form and maintain a good image of Self, which in its turn encourages new undertakings.

The group as Self-object reflects not an exact image, but a beautified one. This is one of the characteristics which distinguish the relationship with a mirror Self-object from Foulkes' 'mirror reaction' which I spoke of in Chapter 1. The authenticity of the image provided by the Mirror Self-object does not rest on the objectivity of realistic judgment, but on the spontaneity of emotional participation. Kohut talks about the glint in a mother's eyes. It is as though the mother or father were saying: 'This is my child, it is the most beautiful child in the world', or 'That is my child walking. Other children can walk, but none are like him. He is fantastic because he can walk.'

When the group has a friendly atmosphere it participates in the victories of each member. Each participant realises that if any of the others takes a step forward, they all move forward. In turn, this leads to an enhancement of positive aspects and shared successes.

The group as a mirror Self-object is often seen as though it were 'almost a person' and shown as such in dreams. For example, Marianna dreams: 'I met a friend of mine and when she came up to me and looked at me ... I felt that I had made contact with the group again.'

Immediately after the group analytic sessions had broken off for the summer holidays, another member of the same group, Aldo, told us: 'Paolo, my music teacher, said goodbye to me. I realised that it was already July, ... I realised that something inside me was breaking. Then I realised that I would miss having someone to listen to what I was learning to play' (see Bejarano 1972; Bion Talamo 1991; Kohut 1971, 1978; Privat and Chapelier 1987; Siani 1992, pp.72–75 and 83).

Technique

In Chapter 3, in dealing with the Fraternal Community stage, I dealt with collective dimensions, and specifically with regard to the group with the emotive cathexis by the participants, and I introduced the notion of the group's affective heritage. Now, I shall consider the problem exclusively from the point of view of the group as a Self-object. First of all, I should like to mention that the three Self-object functions described by Kohut are present in the group. Sometimes the group fulfils the functions of the 'alter ego Self-object' and mirroring Self-object, and the analyst the function of the ideal Self-object. Sometimes the distribution of the functions is different. However, this division is more apparent than real because, as far as this type of experience is concerned, the group and the analyst are seen as a single entity.

The general technical aim is always to respect the Self-object relationship which the members have established with the group. Participants will tolerate a remark regarding one of themselves better than one about the group as a whole. In fact, a remark of this type would touch on something which they imagine and experience as perfect and untouchable (the group) and not something (themselves) which they perceive as limited and needing to evolve. Consequently the analyst needs to avoid judgments of the type 'the group is incapable of dealing with this problem' or 'new ideas are not being brought into the group'. These remarks – even if they give a realistic assessment of the situation – are experienced by the participants in an emotionally amplified way and are seen as a violent and destructive attack. It is very important to take this into account not only in therapeutic groups, but also in groups in which there is a specific task to be carried out. In supervision groups, for example, judgment phantasies are very active, and if the supervisor does not keep a climate of intense and positive affectivity alive, even a minor remark may be seen as a complete disregard of the efforts made and results achieved. This does not mean that the supervisor cannot say what he thinks (falsity is never advantageous); it is only a matter of taking into account the crucial importance of the supervisor's words as a source of mirroring (see Cotinaud 1976; Rogers 1970).

Another indication is that the therapist should participate affectively in the group in a very active way in moments of crisis in the relationship between participants and the group as Self-object. In the therapeutic group we quite often find micro-catastrophes which are actually the result of group analytic work. Demands change, solutions change, phantasies change. One way to make the group function was found, but later it no longer works. It is very important for the therapist to avoid trying to stop change, even if this is experienced as catastrophic. Otherwise it is as though the group were surviving itself as a living group. We might pretend nothing has happened, but a functioning group has become a cult. A working therapist has been transformed into a totem. In the phases when the group is changing its skin, besides enabling the members to recognise the change, as I mentioned, the analyst must accentuate his own affective participation. The analyst's greater affective presence will, on the one hand, supplement the group's Self-object function, and on the other favour the possibility of a renewed cathexis in a transformed group. It is as though the analyst – who increases his participation in moments of crisis – on the one hand fills a void in the relationship created between the participants and the group, and on the other encourages the group's cathexis in its changed position, showing that he is the first to be ready to accept the new situation positively.

A final observation: Freud, but above all Melanie Klein, thought the individual needed to free himself of the group if he were to achieve complete maturity. I share this idea as far as the reduction of conformism and of a tendency to hide behind the anonymity of the group-mass is concerned. However, I would emphasise that for the individual the relationship with the group is a permanent one. The group as a Self-object is essential for his well-being. The loss of group reference, for example, is an extremely important loss. Our aim might be, not to do without the group, but to avoid being bound to just one group, to have the possibility to change, to try out a variety of group situations in the course of our lives.

CHAPTER 17

Effective Narration

In this and the following chapter the theme is not one of the relationship between the group and the individual, but the associated one of the relationship between the group field (common space, semiosphere) and individuals.

Commuting

Pichon-Rivière (1977) observes that a group can effectively deal with the issue of an individual only when it has become an element of the common field, when it has been transformed into 'a configuration which involves the group as a whole'. In other words, transfer, reactivation and registration in the group field are a necessary premise to any useful cognitive and transformative approach to the problems, phantasies and states of mind of the participants. If a phantasy has not entered the field, it will be possible to provide an explanation, propose pedagogic work and build up knowledge about it, but true transformation will not be possible.

Reflecting on the transfer function from the individual sphere to that of the group, which is implicit in Pichon-Rivière's observation, I came up with the expression 'commuter train'. Commuter trains carry passengers daily from one city to another, between suburbs and towns, between residential areas and places of work. A commuter is someone who has a season ticket which allows him to travel from place A to place B and back again.

Dwelling on this word, it seemed to me that it indicated fairly well the to and fro movement between the individual dimension and that of the group. I looked up the verb in the dictionary and saw that it comes from the Latin *cum-mutare*. So, the etymology of the word stresses the fact that a change is made together with others, or rather all together. This feature of the term also corresponds to something important: the change from the individual dimension to that of the group takes place within the group as a whole. In addition there is the fact that, as far as I know, the word has not yet been used in the psychological field and is fairly remote from the term transference, used in traditional (dual) psychoanalysis. I thought, therefore, of suggesting its use – with reference to group analysis – to indicate all those functions which preside over the passage and transformation of elements from the sphere of the individual to that of the group and vice versa.

The question of commuting is very important for various reasons. I shall just touch on two.

- The passage of a theme, an affect, a phantasy from the individual to the group is a premise for the transformation of material in the course of analytic work. An explanation of how this passage takes place will throw some light on an essential aspect of the functioning of the therapeutic factor of group analysis (working through: affective and cognitive transformation) which I spoke about in Chapter 10 (on the therapeutic function of group thought).

- In dealing with this subject it will be possible to highlight analogies and differences between transference (a specific mode of 'transport' in the dual analytic relationship) and the types of passage proper to the group setting.

In this chapter I am going to look, in particular, at the passage from the individual sphere to that of the group and only marginally at the appropriation by the participants of ideas and phantasies worked through by the group. The latter is an important theme to which, however, I shall be able to devote only a few observations in the interview on the therapeutic potentialities of the group, given as an appendix to this book. As far as the analogies and differences between commuting and transference are concerned, I shall simply make a few notes.

From telling a story to becoming a character in it

The passage of thoughts, phantasies and emotions from the individual to the group field can be brought about in various ways which do not form a homogeneous class, but are, on the contrary, profoundly different from each other. Some are voluntary and demand a certain capacity, others are non-voluntary and automatic. An intentional and particularly creative way of commuting is 'effective narration'.

Effective narration is a method of communicating used by group members who are capable of relating a dream, for example, or an episode in their life, in such a way that the other members are led almost spontaneously to associate their phantasies, dreams and thoughts. That is to say, the whole group uses this 'effective narration' for collective work. In my opinion, the analyst should also adopt this means of expression in order to enter into a relationship with the group.

Narrating effectively does not mean describing or representing thoughts or states of mind, but making them interact directly with the people listening and with the elements present in the field. The 'language of effectiveness', as Bion affirms, is not a substitute for action, but has the same immediacy and force. The result of an 'effective narration' is that the facts narrated come to life, and take their place within the living fabric of the group's thought.

Narrating effectively also implies something more than the animation of thoughts and facts. Like a child playing with tin soldiers or cars, it implies that the narrator puts himself into the story.

Vyasa, the author of the great Indian epic poem, *Mahabharata*, like children playing or like members of a group, does not simply tell the story of the Pandavas, but in many key passages of the plot takes an active part, putting himself into relationship with his characters. I mean that he acts not as a *deus ex machina*, but as one of the characters of the narrative fiction. Above all he acts while still remaining himself, Vyasa, the poet. The narrative, that is, becomes another reality in which the author feels, thinks and interacts. For example, when the Pandavas – the heroes of *Mahabharata* – are wandering about aimlessly, they are persuaded by Vyasa to go to Ekacakra, then to the Pancala, where fate intends them to find their wives.

In *A Memoir of the Future* (1975) Bion, too, puts himself into the plot of the book. Or rather, he puts into the narrative many examples of 'himself': Bion, *Myself*, the Psychoanalyst, Captain Bion. These characters, who are the author or one aspect of the author, interact with others who are actual characters.

Conditions necessary for the creation of effective narration

The possibility of 'effective narration' translating into field elements depends on the capacity of whoever is speaking to identify himself with the narrative so as to communicate his emotions and thoughts in extraordinarily intense words and in a genuine and animated way. However, this is not the only condition. In fact, the effectiveness of the narration depends on a number of factors, including:

- A situation of uninterrupted attention. While in the traditional (dual) psychoanalytic situation a precept of fluctuating attention is valid, in the group, 'full attention' is required. What I am alluding to is a state of perceptivity which can pick up a great number of signs of different levels and nature. Nevertheless, this vigilant condition should not be detached from a capacity to listen, at other moments, in a 'fluctuating' and 'receptive' way (see Perri 1993).

- Continually renewed syntony between speaker and listener.

- Intelligence in whoever is listening to the narrative. This function is better expressed by the neologism 'double-think' than by the word 'understand'. In fact, the word 'understand' indicates an affective participation in the experience of the person who is speaking. In speaking of the 'intelligence' of the narrative, on the contrary, I am not seeking to stress this type of participation, but to underline that what must be realised is the real sense of what a person is saying.

The last factor of effective narrative is the requirement that:

• The narrative should be personal, but go beyond an exclusive reference to the speaker's self and his experiences.

The legend of the writing of the *Mahabharata* exemplifies these conditions:

When Vyasa had the whole epic in his mind, he invoked Brahma, the Creator. 'I have composed a magnificent poem.' He explained it to him and asked his help in writing it down. Brahma said: 'Turn to Ganesa. He will be the best one to write down your poem as you recite it.'

Ganesa, the elephant-headed god, accepted the task on condition that there should be no pause in the dictation. The author accepted, provided that Ganesa received and understood the meaning of every single word before putting it into writing.

Vyasa dictated at an incredible speed, but Ganesa kept up with him, transcribing most zealously. When at a certain point his pen broke, he snapped off one of his tusks and used it to go on writing. Every now and then the author realised that his scribe was beating him in speed, and he slowed him down by composing here and there dense and sententious passages which obliged Ganesa to stop writing in order to reflect on their meaning.

Sprechgesang

I shall add a few more words on this last condition, which is necessary if an intervention is to become effective narration. As I have pointed out, this condition is that it must go beyond what is only and exclusively the narrator's experience or personal feeling. That is, it must contain and express, besides personal experience, the emotions and phantasies present in the group at that moment. Only if the life of the whole group is expressed in the narrative, is it really possible for the other participants to see in it, alongside the experiences of the speaker, something which belongs to them. It is this possibility which enables the other members to intervene by association, bringing in dreams, phantasies and thoughts. By this I do not mean that whoever is speaking should be the group spokesperson. Neither do I mean that effective narration must have the emotions and phantasies present in the group as its object. I mean that these should be contained in a synthetic and syncopated form. To explain myself better, I shall use an analogy taken from the world of music.

The German expression *Sprechgesang* (that is, sung speech) does not indicate a type of technique or performance corresponding to the recitative of Italian opera. In recitative the notes are intoned regularly; the difference from singing lies only in the fact that the melodic lines and motifs are never very elaborate or developed.

The *Sprechgesang*, which was introduced by Schonberg and first used by him in *Pierrot Lunaire* and *Moses und Aaron* to restore dignity and specificity to the reciting voice, consists instead of uttering the note shown in the score only at the beginning of the speech; this note is then rendered into spoken words. (see Santi 1989, pp.734–735).

In the same way, effective intervention picks up the note that prevails in the group at the moment of intervention and then carries on with the narrative 'holding' the note. The whole path that whoever is speaking has followed, in order to bring to light the emotive and phantasmatic context, is synthesised in the first note. To be more precise, this is the path he has had to follow to present in reality the emotive and phantasmatic context which exists in the session, which up to that moment could not be brought to light. This is an operation which requires a lot of time and effort, but when it is carried out it is done rapidly. A brief clinical illustration will enable me to clarify this aspect of the subject.

> Right from the beginning of the session, those who speak, one after the other seem to want to force group involvement through an escalation of emotional tone. The desired involvement in participation, however, does not appear. Elisa, for example, leans forward several times as though she were about to speak, then remains silent. A brief discussion takes place between some of those present, in which doubt is cast on the effectiveness of the animated narration of facts that are more and more miraculous and stupefying in an effort to make the group function well. Immediately afterwards, Maria Giovanna, in a subdued tone which contrasts with the tone and the exertion of the first part of the session, says in a soft and rather plaintive voice that on her way to the group, she had been in a playful mood, then when the session began she had become dull. She goes on to narrate some of her thoughts and phantasies. Elisa, as though Maria Giovanna had set her off on the right note, tells of a recent episode in which she was rejected and not understood by her husband. Fedia adds to what Maria Giovanna and Elisa have said, that today she feels slow and sleepy. The group's situation is now receptive, controlled pain can be sensed. There is a completely different atmosphere from the animated and high-flying one which they were trying to produce at the beginning of the session; but now everyone present is taking part in the discussion, both men and women.

> Just as in *Sprechgesang*, Maria Giovanna – with her submissive and plaintive tone of voice, and by referring to the change in her state of mind when she entered the group – picked up the 'low tone' of the emotions which were really present in the group. This enabled Elisa and Fedia to speak, and then the group as a whole was able to start working together again.

Unsaturated interpretation

There is another point about *Sprechgesang*. As I said before, this technique particularly interested me because the melody is summarised in a punctiform manner in
the way the first note is sung, and it appeared to me a useful instrument for developing some of the possible articulations between the group and the themes which
are present, but still unexpressed, in the group. I examined this problem in Chapters 1 and 8 when I dealt with the star-shape, mimesis and 'unison' with 'O'. Soavi
(1989) suggests something similar with regard to the formulation of interpretations. It is perhaps possible to speak of interpretations which, rather than put into
words, are given in an empathetic response. The analyst, for example, intervenes
in the analysand's discourse with participatory sounds such as 'mmmm!!!' or with
interjections which have the function of accentuating the sense of what the analysand is saying: '...ah!!!'. On other occasions he repeats one or more of the words
spoken by the analysand: 'the dog??!!' '...in the country house...'. 'Interpretations without words' seek to pick up an emotion present at that moment and to
provide the mirror effect that the analysand is waiting for without extending the
verbal and argumentative part of the analyst's intervention, which is almost completely absent.

E. Gaburri and E. Contardi (1993) offer another useful contribution to the
relationship between *Sprechgesang* and interpretation. They suggest that it is its
non-saturation characteristic which is capable of opening up interpretation in
order that the members of the group can bring in their dreams and phantasies by
association. The idea, contained both in my suggestion of summarising the entire
melodic line in one intonation and in the suggestion of leaving the interpretation
unsaturated, is that effective intervention sets the group on the right track, but is
not a substitute for working through and transforming.

Gaburri and Contardi also add a few other observations which relate to interpretation, but can also be extended to any effective narration. They write that
interpretation, if it is to become a truly transforming factor, besides receiving and
working through repressed or split-off elements, needs to be unsaturated in order
to take a position and act effectively within the transpersonal emotive group field.
The non-saturation of an intervention derives from awareness that interpretive
language may be inadequate and must therefore be integrated with what is unsaid
yet present in the emotive group field – something unsaid which is as yet unspeak-
able because the symbolic elements for communicating it verbally have not been
formed. It follows then that unsaturated interpretation exposes both the group
and the individual to a certain state of malaise because, while it relieves the need to
know, it also arouses feelings of persecution, due to maintaining in the field
unknown elements that could develop in unpredictable ways.

Therefore, in effective narration there will always be elements, like *Sprechgesang*
or non-saturation, which cannot yet be fully expressed. They will constitute the

future themes of the group, and space will be left for the existence of other rhythms, other points of view, which may be different from those of the speaker.

CHAPTER 18

Transtemporal Diffusion

I shall continue the argument of the previous chapter by examining another method of commuting between individual and group. Effective narration, as we have seen, is an intentional way of commuting, which demands an effective expressive capacity. On the other hand, the type of commuting of which I am now about to speak takes place without the individual being aware of it, but rather by means of him. For this form I have chosen the name 'transtemporal diffusion'.

The word 'diffusion' indicates that this is not a 'transport' or a passage, but a silent occupation of the group's field. We could imagine the diffusion of a gas which cannot be stopped in any way by the barriers represented by the group or the 'psychic skin' of individuals.

The other word, 'transtemporal' indicates that the diffusion can even occur between individuals and groups who are distant in space and time; for example, between the participant's family of origin, or an institution where he lived as a child, and the group field. Diffusion is also possible through several generations of a family: trans-generational diffusion. I shall note in passing that we have already taken into consideration some aspects of transtemporality, with reference to the transtemporality of 'mental fields' mentioned in Chapter 13.

What is habitually transmitted by transtemporal diffusion is a sort of 'being together', a certain way of seeing oneself. I do not think we should speak of the diffusion of 'fields', but that we should refer with greater precision to the diffusion of specific qualities of the field. For example, boredom, which reigned in the family and kept it united, or a quality of noble suffering which coloured every act, or lies and hypocrisy which permeated every relationship and every thought. In certain cases I have had the impression that what was diffused was not a characteristic but more a spell or enchantment like the one which sent Sleeping Beauty's castle to sleep.

The result of the diffusion of these 'elements' is that two fields which may be very different – for example, the field of the patient's family of origin and the group field – have one or more common (invariant) elements and are therefore similar in a certain sense.

Here is a clinical example to show what I mean by enchantment. It is the phantasy of a very young girl, capable of strong intuitions and also of representing her own states of mind and those of the group in a plastic way. Her phantasy was told in an analytic group and gives a representation of the patient's family field and the field which has been established in the group through transtemporal diffusion. To understand the sense of the phantasy, some preliminary information is necessary.

> Right from the beginning of the analysis, Graziella has regularly brought to the group stories of the dramatic vicissitudes of her sister, whose asocial and sometimes openly violent behaviour worried her constantly.

> Some weeks ago the situation changed because Graziella's sister decided to undergo treatment, left the family and was now living abroad, in a Latin American country. In the sessions after telling the group this news Graziella no longer mentions her sister.

> There follows a period during which Graziella is very active in the group, attracting attention to herself and also setting up a certain amount of violence and intimidation. The therapist and the other members succeed in confronting this behaviour without excessive conflicts and in creating conditions for overcoming the situation which has arisen in the group.

> I shall now refer more directly to the events of the session during which Graziella narrates the phantasy I mentioned earlier.

> The theme of the first part of the session is 'expressing one's own thoughts, phantasies and states of mind'. Gianna – who speaks immediately before Graziella – says she has grown fond of her (Gianna's) bad moods, hates and grudges. Expressing them would be a little like losing them. Gianna is especially afraid that if she expressed herself she would finish up as empty as a sack. Graziella picks up Gianna's intervention, saying that while she was listening to the other people this image was conjured up in her mind; 'as though a thread came out of the mouths of those who were expressing their thoughts. The threads went from the mouth of one person to the mouth of another. What was expressed was a thickening of the thread, a little being. These little beings, coming out of their mouths, remained suspended in the net and died of starvation'.

> Graziella's phantasy represents interpersonal relationships (the threads which go from the mouth of one to the mouth of another) and the field (the net).

> The spell which falls on the group is this: no one takes up the words to give a syntonic reflection to the person who has expressed her state of mind. Even the field does not nourish or protect or give warmth.

> The stimulation to speak and seek contact – associated with negation and refusal – forms an image which, in a certain sense, is perverse. The needs (the little beings) remain suspended in mid-air: they are not separated from those who

have spoken and not received by those who should have responded. So they die slowly of hunger and abandonment.

The agony of the little beings who die in the field of Graziella's family of origin, because neither individuals nor the environment are interested in them or capable of giving them life, is diffused within the group as squalor, violence and conflict. The group and the analyst, according to Graziella's experience, are also showing themselves to be incapable of creating a truly alternative situation.

Graziella, when painfully relating this phantasy, is trying to give her contribution to overcoming the situation which has arisen.

Technique

There are three general considerations:

The first can be expressed in these terms: the elements which are transtemporally diffused often have viral characteristics in that they use the forces of the host, in this case the group, to distort communication. Rancour, desperation and guilt, for example, do not only use their own forces, but multiply them through polarisation of the group's 'mental field', which excludes the mitigating presence of other feelings. The diffuse element – in the case of another patient who lived for a long time in an institution – was an extremely pervasive feeling of cold which was transmitted through the inevitable transformation of the group's conversation into an abstract discussion.

The second consideration relates to the totalising tendency of the diffuse elements with regard to the group field. I should emphasise that their effectiveness depends on the achievement of complete or almost complete saturation of the field. Boredom and depression, for example, increase their power by almost completely impregnating the 'field' of intelligence and imagination.

- What is diffused is often something that up to that moment showed up only as an obscure zone of experience or as an element of rigidity of self; a dense hypercomplex field in which what is personal and what belongs to the family, the clan, the group, is confused.

- The break-up of the pathological personal-family nucleus is sometimes evidenced by the appearance of symptoms or experiences of loss. These must be seen as a consequence of the patient's attempt to free himself of the conditions in which he finds himself.

- The diffusion of 'pathological qualities' in the analytic field is a moment in which the patient tries, with the help of the analyst and the other members, to face up to something which up to then he has had to deal with alone.

These considerations give rise to some technical suggestions:

- It is indispensable for the analyst to strive to keep the various dimensions and functions of the analytic field active and lively in order to avoid its collapse.

- The analyst and the group must not use sudden breaks in order to emerge from the pathological field, but, on the contrary, they must proceed by small adjustments so as not to lose that contact which was first made possible by pathology and suffering, and which is essential for the patient who has transmitted the pathological field to the group. When the 'pathological field' has been destructured, at least in part, and made more ductile, the analyst will be able to describe, to this member and the other participants, a field whose characteristics will allow them to be aware of life, emotion and thought.

Appendices

At the end of this book there still remain some very relevant themes to be dealt with:

- the psychological condition of the mass
- the process of institutionalisation of the group
- the therapeutic value of group analysis.

Detailed treatment of these subjects would almost mean writing a second volume; yet not mentioning them would deprive the book of something essential. I have tried to solve this problem by presenting this part of the book in the form of an interview, which enables me to present ideas in a synthetic and incisive way. The two first interviews were given to Marco Zanori, the third to Stefania Marinelli. I wish to thank them for their contribution to the presentation and investigation of the themes we have discussed.

The Group and the Psychological Mass
Interview with M. Zanori

M.Z.: *What are the characteristics of the psychological condition of mass in the small analytic group?*

C.N.: In certain circumstances, in the small group, there is a sort of agglutination between those present and the emotional situation. To clarify what I mean, I shall refer to the dream of a patient who belonged to an analytic group. In the dream of this patient, who is called Sandro, the agglutination is represented as a mixture. 'I came into the room used by the group: all the walls were covered with a non-figurative painting, there were colours and masses, but no figure. It was not a picture, but rather a fresco; the painting was done directly on the walls, and there were frames on them, but only placed over them. In some areas this unformed picture had greater coherence and acquired a certain structure; it was as though it were trying to come away from the wall and go out towards the door of the room. I was in the room with another three or four people from the group and the analyst; it seemed to me that the others were laughing at these attempts to get out of the mass.'

The cohesion of the group, transformed into a mass according to what is shown in the images in Sandro's dream, is obtained through loss of distinction between the figures, and by their convergence in an almost fluid emotional and sensorial condition.

Sandro's dream also defines, in a psychological sense, some of the motivations of the group as a mass: common defence, search for anonymity, fear of derision and envy. We can also recognise the efforts of some members to find (or recover) an embryonic identity, for instance in that part of the dream in which some areas of the fresco where the unformed painting is shown to be acquiring greater coherence and structure.

M.Z.: *The image of the mass of colours painted directly on the wall brings to my mind a dream mentioned in a book by Charlotte Beradt. Charlotte Beradt is concerned with the years in Germany just before the Nazis came to power. In order to develop her work, Beradt uses an unusual historio-graphical method: dreams.*

The dream which came to my mind when you were telling me about the picture without frames was that of a doctor. In his dreams these are the images which appeared: 'When my visits are finished, about nine at night, I am on the point of lying down quietly on the divan with a book, when suddenly the walls of my room and my flat disappear. I look around in consternation; all the flats that I can see no longer have any walls. I hear a loudspeaker blaring: in accordance with the decree of the 17th of the month, relating to the removal of walls ...'

In the dream of your patient, Sandro, there are coloured masses which no longer have frames. The doctor whose dream is mentioned by Charlotte Beradt seems to me to be terrified of the risk of a collapse of his 'mental-walls skin'. I should like to ask you this: is the loss of boundaries an essential moment in the creation of the mass? Can it be expressed in terms of a threat to the integrity of that function which E. Bick calls 'mental skin' and D. Anzieu calls 'skin-Ego'?

C.N.: When the group-mass is constituted there is a rapid and violent movement of the boundary function – the mental skin, the skin-Ego – which passes from the individual to the group as a whole. I shall again use a few images. In fact, the effects of this displacement of the boundary function of the 'mental skin' are effectively represented in a phantasy expressed by another participant, Luigi, in the course of a session following shortly after the one in which Sandro related his dream.

In this phantasy, the group is imagined as a swarming mass, but it is in some way bounded. This is the phantasy related by Luigi: 'I thought of a book which had impressed me some time ago; it described how, in a given circumstance, the whole earth was covered with a carpet of swarming flies 20 to 50 cm high. I thought then that the essential function was that of the flies on the surface: the thickness of the carpet was not very important because the other flies were controlled by those above them.'

Every fly, every single element of the mass probably corresponds to an 'individual-member' or the parts held in common by different individual-members. It is also possible to hypothesise that the elements of the mass of flies correspond to perceptions and feelings which have been aroused. Even if the boundaries of the individuals and those between single individuals are indefinite and continually changing, the boundaries of the whole system begin to acquire a structure. The more evolved elements come to the surface and fulfil a function of self-containment (even of concealment) for the more primitive elements; there is no real distinction between contained and container, but rather a stratification thanks to which the contained produces a kind of container.

M.Z.: If a group is to be transformed into a group-mass, is it important for a systematic attack to be made on the 'private space of Self'?

C.N.: These attacks are of great importance, but many different factors are involved in the activation within the group of the psychological condition of mass. Another relevant factor is the presence of a tyrannical leader. If the leader suppresses the expression of the members' thoughts by constant criticism, the group remains at a low level of mental development. The only 'thought' is that of the leader, the other members echo his thought.

M.Z.: Petrolini represents the relationship between the tyrant-leader and the mass as a pseudo-playful child's mirror-game: a relationship of love sensations. Nero, the charismatic leader, after himself causing the burning of Rome, declaimed emphatically and pompously: 'I shall rebuild a Rome more beautiful than ever!!!' The mass applauds. The charismatic leader, delighted, repeats the phrase with greater emphasis: 'I shall rebuild a Rome more beautiful ...' The mass applauds harder and more rapidly. 'I shall rebuild a Rome ...' Applause. 'I shall rebuild ...' Applause. 'I shall ...' Thunder of applause. 'Rome ...' Thunder of enthusiastic applause. At the end the leader says only a fragment of a word: 'Ro ...' He says nothing. And the applause comes at once. The applause precedes the words. It becomes a struggle. The vain dictator cannot speak, the mass applauds him before he opens his mouth.

C.N.: The mass and the tyrant devour each other.

M.Z.: *Do the mutual devouring of the leader and the group and the pulling down of the barriers of the single individuals derive from a common factor?*

C.N.: I would say there is relevance in the emergence of the need to look at (and pretend to experience) 'strong emotions' and 'pure emotions'. I use this expression in the sense in which it is used for colours: it is said of some colours that they are 'pure colours'. Yellow is a pure colour, because it is not produced by the mixing of other colours.

'Pure emotions' are not combined with other emotions; they are devouring because they cancel out other feelings. Terror can be defined as a pure emotion because it tends to invade the entire field of the group. Extreme idealisation works in the same way. This invasive monoculture finishes by bringing down the leader, the group and the persons taking part in it.

M.Z.: *'Pure emotion', if I have understood properly, creates a very powerful common zero setting which annuls individuality, transforming any number of people into a group-mass.*

C.N.: Yes, certain mental states have a very appealing power.

M.Z.: *As I listened to you, I began to think of Nazism, and Gunther Grass's book 'The Tin Drum' came to mind. The main character of the book is a child, who is also the only character who succeeds in remaining outside the great Nazi assemblies. The child with the tin drum does not want to grow up; not growing up is his way of escaping the Nazi masses, the hypnotic reign of pure emotions, the alienating surrender of the most free and creative aspect of his identity, which would inevitably follow his entry into adulthood.*

C.N.: The problem of all participants in a group is that of growing up, which means becoming a full member of a group without losing oneself. In other words, what must prevail is the bringing to the fore of individual and collective responsibility rather than the idea of 'group-mass'.[1]

---

1   For further reading see: Beradt, C. (1966) Bick, E. (1968) Anzieu, D. (1985); Khan, M.M.R. (1974); Petrolini (1917); Grass, G. (1990); Amati Sas, S. (1977); Bettelheim, B. (1966); Canetti, E. (1960) In C. Neri *et al.* (1991); Freud, S. (1912–13) and Freud, S. (1921).

The Transformation of a Group into an Institution
Interview with M. Zanori

M.Z. A famous passage in Dostoevsky depicts an imaginary meeting and dispute between Christ and the Grand Inquisitor. The action takes place in Spain, when the Inquisition is at its height. During a 'grandiose auto-da-fé,' Christ appears and they all (how strange!) recognise him. The Cardinal in person, the Grand Inquisitor, orders the guards to arrest him. They take Christ to prison. At the end of the day the old Grand Inquisitor goes alone into the prison. He looks into the face of Christ and says to him: 'Why have you come? You refused the only path which could lead men to bliss. The great spirit, the Devil, spoke to you in the wilderness. He asked you three questions. Remember the first one: "You see these stones? Turn them into bread, and humanity will follow you, with dignity and in obedience." But you refused the suggestion. Where would freedom be, you reasoned, if consent could be bought with bread? But this very request for a common genuflection has been the greatest torment of every single man and of humanity as a whole since the beginning of time. The terrible and very wise spirit, the Devil, took you to the summit of the Temple and said, "If you want to know whether you are the Son of God, throw yourself down." You realised that by making the slightest movement, you would have challenged the Lord, and you would then have lost all the faith you had in him. But is human nature perhaps made in such a way that, in the most terrible, heart-rending moments of life, the ones most deeply demanding of the soul, it can still stay true to a free decision of the heart? We have emended your acts, and men are delighted to be once more led like a flock of sheep.'

Here Dostoevsky, in my opinion, illustrates how the suggestion of a new idea or the detailed re-reading of an original idea, represented by Jesus' return, can reactivate expectation and hope in the group, but also create turbulence and the experience of a persecution which has been sedated and controlled by the Institution. In particular, Dostoevsky shows how the impulse towards change meets not only the opposition of the Institution, from the Grand Inquisitor, but also from the group, whose members desire a common genuflection. It is as though they said: 'We emerged with great difficulty from the turbulence and emotional tumult brought about by Christ's new idea. It was a difficulty which was useful, but to go back to that condition, which we had such trouble getting away from, is painful and almost unbearable.'

Does something analogous also happen in the small psycho-analytic group?

C.N.: In the small group there is no organisation or hierarchy, but all the same it may tend to become like a little community. The members not only share values, aspirations and emotions, but they do also institutionalise them. They acquire a feeling of existence and security from the boundaries of the group to which they belong and the confirmation of its values.

M.Z.: This corresponds to the Institution, to the Grand Inquisitor, so what of the second, Messianic function, represented by Christ?

C.N.: In the small analytic group there are intense Messianic impulses. However, the important thing is not so much their presence as the fact that they are linked up with psychoanalysis, that is to say with a method and research which is aimed at knowing oneself through direct experience, in a one-to-one relationship or in a group.

On this subject I should like to speak about an 'experience-function' of the small analytic group. This function corresponds to the analytic task of the group, which is to look at phantasies and emotions, bring out internal tensions, and pass from events to experience. 'Learning from experience' is essential if development and change are to occur.

M.Z.: *On the other hand, does the organisation of the group as a little community, which I should like to define as an 'institution-function', represent a flight of the members of the group away from themselves and their experiences?*

C.N.: I would not see the 'institution-function' and the 'experience-function' as being in direct opposition. The path and the aims which we seek to attain through group analysis are very different from those which are sought for example by a therapeutic community, although participation in this type of community is often accompanied by substantial therapeutic results.

M.Z.: *Do you mean that the institution-function and the experience-function are complementary?*

C.N.: Cohesion and stability, which are proper to the institution-function, constitute a necessary support for the cognitive and analytic functions of the group. However, too vigorous a development of the institution-function may obstruct the working of analytic functions. For example, members of the group may be led to prefer stability to knowledge and consider that participation in the group does not count, that it is enough to be 'a faithful follower of psycho-analysis' to achieve a cure. One characteristic of the analytic group, therefore, is to limit the 'institutional aspects' of the group and to exploit, on the other hand, its thinking and working-through functions.

M.Z: *What can the analyst of the group do to encourage the development of the experience-function and limit that of the institution-function?*

C.N.: He should not repeat slogans and catchwords, and he should avoid favouring the tendency to stabilise the network of relationships in fixed roles. The analyst must also try to revive feelings which have become conventional, energising group situations which have become crystallised. All this should be done delicately and in a respectful way: for example, by encouraging the possibility of a new perspective on experience or by giving space to an underlying emotion which is usually left to one side.

M.Z.: *Is this essentially a mental attitude?*

C.N.: To be effective, every intervention of the analyst must come from his inner mind and act first of all on himself. To limit the development of the institution-function, for example, the analyst must first of all separate himself from some aspects of his own personality which need the support of general agreement; 'It is not enough to have distanced ourselves from people; we must also distance ourselves from the inclinations which are common to all of us; we must cut ourselves off from ourselves."[1]

---

[1]   Dostoevsky's text quoted in the interview is taken from Dostoevsky (1880) *The Brothers Karamazov*. The second quotation appearing in the interview is from Montaigne, M. (1957). Other books and articles, even if not directly quoted, are important for the direction of the argument: Bauman, Z. (1989) ; Bion, W.R. (1961) Bion, W.R. (1970); De Lillo, D. (1991) Cinciripini, C. and Di Leone, G. (1990); Jaffé R. (1992).

Therapeutics in the Group
Interview with S. Marinelli

S.M.: *Does group analysis offer patients the possibility of escaping from the isolation neurosis places them in?*

C.N.: For people taking part in analysis, entering the world of the group – a world which is seen especially in the initial phases, as rather different from the one in which their problems emerged, represents an experience on which their whole interest is centred. Consequently, at the beginning of therapy the majority of participants concentrate on the task of entering into relationship with the group and with the other members, rather than their need to talk about their own problems. When the group begins participants often do not speak of their problems at all. Then when the moment comes to present their problems, they can be placed and considered within the weaving fabric of thoughts and group relationships which have been built up in the meantime.

S.M.: *Can the expression 'escaping from isolation' also have some other meaning besides that of participating in this new 'group' situation group?*

C.N.: In the group, the patients discover – sometimes to their amazement – that certain difficulties and fears which they thought were exclusively theirs are on the contrary common to all or to the majority of those present. This discovery frees them, at least partly, from feelings of shame which have been with them for years. I might add that there is often a dominant phantasy at the source of this feeling of shame: the phantasy of 'being a monster', or that there is a part of them that is monstrous.

S.M.: *With this idea of being a monster we are approaching another theme which I should like to discuss with you. And it is this: does a group psychoanalytical experience orientate the development of identity?*

C.N.: In the group it is easier to perceive the idea of one's own identity as being multiple. Multiplicity, understood not as a transitory moment, but on the contrary as the basis of identity. In my opinion, in fact, the group constitutes a sort of model of 'functioning multiplicity', not only because of the presence of several people, but also of the multifaceted and global aspects of its thought.

S.M.: *What other identity characteristics are encouraged by group analysis?*

C.N.: When analysis achieves good results, there is a feeling of openness and enrichment, thanks to being in a relationship with an object which is perceived as being endowed with great power and fecundity. This recalls the legends of heroes raised not by a woman but by a wild animal. In the most successful cases, this feeling is associated with the attribution of less importance to personal success than to the success of common projects. The members of an analytic group experience their positive fulfilment as taking place within the context of the overall progress of the group and never to the detriment of the other members.

S.M.: *Is the feeling, experienced by the members of the group, that analysis brings about a transformation, not only of themselves as single individuals but also of the group as a whole, a characteristic which distinguishes group analysis from one-to-one analysis?*

C.N.: Yes, it is. In fact, in the group the transformation concerns not only individuals, but also the group itself, which ceases to be a 'waste land' and becomes fertile. In other words, in the small analytic group, the phantasy and the experience of being cured involve not only the participants, but also the regeneration of the group as a whole. It is impossible to imagine a group in which the participants are cured while the group remains sterile.

S.M.: *Does group analysis encourage the analysand to be more active than they would be in the dual setting?*

C.N.: It becomes clear fairly early on that every participant receives in relation to what he invests in work is common. Self-promotion is a must in the group situation. An old Chinese tradition comes to mind: immediately after birth the newborn baby is placed on the ground and left there. This is so that it will make contact with the forces of the great Earth-mother, but above all so that in calling and crying it can give its first sign of vitality and active demands. At this point it is welcomed and given its first name.

Similarly, in group analysis it is essential for the individual to give a sign that he wishes to be welcomed and helped by the group. When he has done this, his right to exist and to have an emotional and relational space is recognised. Later on he will become capable of recognising this right for himself.

S.M.: *How does this recognition come about?*

C.N. The analyst points out the elements of difference and individuality of the single participants in the group: the characteristics of their thought and their style. He also responds to their emerging competences. For example, he shows that he has seen and confirms the existence of certain new capacities of the individual, allowing him to make them his own.

S.M.: *Has the importance given to individual characteristics and the discovery of competences anything to do with the acquisition of awareness of one's own identity?*

C.N.: They are different moments. The acquisition of awareness of one's own identity is more complex. Moreover, awareness of our own identity is attained by considering ourselves more from a historical and retrospective than from a prospective point of view. According to Melanie Klein, awareness of self gains consistency in a depressive situation: that is to say, at the moment when the individual has the possibility of reflecting and looking back; in these depressive moments, it is easier for him to collect his thoughts together and accept the experience of his life, and realise what his limitations are.

S.M.: *In what other way can we become aware of our own identity during analytic work?*

C.N.: By separating self from the phantasies which keep us from recognising ourselves. Speaking of analytic work, Freud uses the metaphor of sculpture. Sculpture, unlike painting, is a work which implies taking away, digging out and not one of laying on.

S.M.: *With regard to this work of self-recognition, can the group also have the negative effect of adding illusory and saturating elements?*

C.N.: Certainly. Here the analyst's work is one of counteracting. For example, the members of the group, at least at the beginning of analysis, tend rather to fill in, to live entirely within a single homogeneous emotion. The danger of this kind of procedure is that some individual problems can remain unseen.

S.M.: *How did you come to realise that this danger existed?*

C.N.: Some patients, years after the end of their group analysis, have come back to me to tell me about some event in their life, for example marriage or the birth of a child. A certain number of these patients had benefited from their intense participation in the group, and in general the analysis had been a success, but I realised that some of their 'nuclei of suffering' had remained suspended in the gravitational field of the group without ever completely coming down to earth.

S.M.: *What do you mean by nuclei of suffering?*

C.N.: I am not referring to the basic problem for which they had sought analysis, but to some other aspect of their experience which had not been adequately worked through. Sometimes the residual suffering of these patients was encysted in certain silent aspects of their relationship with me, their analyst.

S.M.: *What has this fact suggested to you from the point of view of leading a group?*

C.N.: I have tried to pay more attention to the problem of how to relate the 'private' dimension of the relationship which members of a group have with me, as the therapist, to that 'of the group'. Foulkes, on this subject, speaks of 'configuration'. According to Foulkes, even when something seems to exclusively concern the relationship between a participant and the analyst, a 'configuration' can always be found which shows how the question also concerns the group as a whole.

S.M.: *Returning to the nuclei of suffering which remain 'in orbit', I should like to ask whether in your opinion everything should be included in the field of analysis?*

C.N.: No, but it is painful when there is something which we have never, absolutely never, spoken about with anybody, something which nobody knows.[1]

---

1   The testimony on the Chinese custom of laying the newborn baby on the ground is taken from Granet, M. (1922); Lugones, M. (1994) Some other books and articles, even if not directly quoted in the interview, are essential references to the argument which is developed in the conversation: Ammaniti, M. and Fraire, M. (1982); Bauleo, A. (1974); Di Chiara, G. (1992); Manfredi Turillazzi, S. (1974); Mobasser, E. (1992); Petrini, R. (1986).

Glossary

Various reasons have led me to add a glossary. The first is to provide in a synthetic form some of the original notions suggested in this book. For example: 'Emerging state of the group' and 'commuting'. The second is to specify the sense of some words which are used with a meaning that differs either from that of daily life or from that which is usual in a psychological and psychiatric environment. The words 'Institution' which I use in accordance with the definition of W.R. Bion, and 'Immaterial similarity' which is a specific reference to the thought of W. Benjamin, are prototypes. The third reason is a general one. It is easier for me to explain it with an image. In a wood, no plant could live without the presence and proximity of the innumerable vegetable and animal species which form its habitat. Similarly, ideas need to interact with other thoughts, concepts and images. This glossary is an attempt to form the richest possible habitat for the ideas contained in this book. It is a collection of words which correspond to all those terms, concepts and notions, whose presence in the book seemed to me essential, even if for various reasons I could not explain them in the text. Every entry in the Glossary, as will be seen, is accompanied by a synthetic bibliographical indication. When I prepared these indications I preferred books to articles appearing in specialised reviews. The reason is a practical one: for anyone wishing to study in greater detail the themes dealt with in the glossary, books are easier to obtain. I should add that the bibliographical indications appearing in the glossary include those shown in the text of the book and in the general bibliography.

Adhesive Identification (E. Bick): If the containing function is not adequately carried out by the mother, or is damaged by destructive phantasy attacks of the baby itself, it is not introjected; normal introjection is replaced by the continual use of pathological projective identification which causes identity confusion. States of 'non-integration' persist. The baby frantically seeks an object – light, voice, odour etc. – which will allow it to maintain a unifying attention to the parts of its body, permitting, at least temporarily, the experience of keeping together the parts of Self. It also keeps itself together through the relationship with these objects, and especially by 'adhering', 'being stuck' to the mother. Associated Notions: Character armour, Ego-skin, Mental skin. Essential Bibliography: Bick, E. (1968) *The Experience of the Skin in Early Object-relations.* Tavistock Publications, London.

Affective Heritage of the Group: A series of elements cathected with affects form part of the 'affective heritage of the group': the completeness of the group, the continuity of the sessions, the history of the group, the good functioning of the group and the good impression it makes. An essential characteristic of the 'Affective heritage of the group' is the bi-directionality of the affective currents. The members cathect the group with affects, and the group makes an important contribution to the identity and well-being of its members. This aspect of the function of the Affective heritage of the group is directly related to its function as Self-object. Associated Notions: Original mythical contract, Group as Self-object, World of It, Nomos. Essential Bibliography: Searles, H.F. (1960) *The Non-Human Environment.* Karnac Books, London.

Analysis in Groups: See under *Group analytical psychotherapy* in the Glossary.

Analytic Space: Analytic space, according to Viderman (1970) 'is at the same time a place in the physical world and an imaginary place...where the analytic process will find all its strength and develop all its possibilities'. Corrao (1977 and 1982) describes it as: 'a changeable context able to produce cognitive constructions in expansion by means of expressive plans or projects...which are structured either in speech or in interpretation'. In this book, the 'analytic space' is considered as a dimension of the 'common space' of the small analytic group. Associated Notions: Semiosphere, Common space of the group. Essential Bibliography: Lucas, P. (1985) 'L'espace analytique des groupes thérapeutiques.' *Revue de psychothérapie psycho-analytique 1–2*, 119–133; Viderman, S. (1970) *La construction de l'espace analytique.* Gallimard, Paris, 1982.

Animation: Animation is the process through which, in the course of group therapy, certain capacities of a person, which up to that moment had remained a potential, take on consistency. Animation is produced by the conjunction of two factors. The intensity of emotive participation which distinguishes group life, and the presence within it of ways of thinking which are very different from those which are proper to a participant's family and the world from which he comes. Associated Notions: Initiation. Essential Bibliography: Pasolini, P.P. (1956) *Le ceneri di Gramsci.* Einaudi, Turin.

Anomie (E. Durkheim): E. Durkheim (1897) uses this term to express an absence of values due to the collapse of stable social and family norms in contemporary cities. By the rule of opposites, this concept shows up the individual's need for structural relationships, objects of identification and roles which enable him to see that he is within an understandable frame of reference and consequently to realise that he is safe. Associated Notions: Seriality. Essential Bibliography: Durkheim, E. (1897) *Suicide: A Study in Sociology.* Kegan Paul, London, 1952.

Anti-Group: The exotic, which was an important category of nineteenth-century bourgeois mentality, corresponded in a very limited way to the conditions of life of those populations considered as being exotic. Similarly the anti-group of the small analytic group is neither an enemy nor friendly nor alien group but essentially an aspect of group identity which is experienced by attributing its characteristics to another group. Associated Notions: Self-representation, Boundaries of the group. Essential Bibliography: Lotman, J.M. (1978) *Universe of the Mind.* Bloomington, IN: Indiana University Press.

Artificial Masses (S. Freud): Freud distinguishes between 'primitive masses' and 'artificial masses' (for example, the army and the church) The latter are more stable and are preserved from disintegration by the presence of a leader, by an internal articulation and also by a certain degree of constriction which is exerted on its components in order to prevent them from breaking away. Freud's distinction shows that the psychological condition of mass may be a stable form of social organisation, rather than a transitory condition. Associated Notions: Mass, Totalitarian mass. Essential Bibliography: Freud, S. (1921) *Group Psychology and the Analysis of the Ego.* SE XVIII.

Attachment (J. Bowlby): Bowlby defines attachment as the condition in which the individual is emotionally linked to another person who is seen as being stronger and wiser than himself. The proof of the existence of a relationship of attachment is in the seeking of proximity between two individuals and the phenomenon of the 'secure base'. When he is certain of having a 'secure base' the weaker, smaller person is able to explore his environment. Another proof of the existence of a bond of attachment is the protest expressed upon separation. Associated Notions: Self-object. Essential Bibliography: Bowlby, J. (1969) *Attachment and Loss.* Vol 1, *Attachment.* Hogarth Press, London, 1982; Bowlby, J. (1988) *A Secure Base. Clinical Applications of the Attachment Theory.* Routledge, London; Holmes, J. (1993) *John Bowlby: An Attachment Theory.* Routledge, London.

Attachment Theory. Routledge, London; Holmes, J. (1993) *John Bowlby: An Attachment Theory.* Routledge, London.

Attunement: See note p.89. Associated Notions: Resonance. Essential Bibliography: Correale, A. (1991) *Il campo istituzionale.* Borla, Rome.

Background Tone (F. Redl): See glossary entry *Group atmosphere.*

Basic Assumptions (W.R. Bion): 'Group mentality' is the common, unanimous and anonymous opinion of the group at a given moment. The concept of basic assumption tells us something about the content of this 'group mentality'. Basic assumption of dependence: the group has the secret and unconscious conviction of being met together so that someone on whom the group depends in an absolute way can satisfy all its needs and desires. Basic assumption of fight–flight: the dominant phantasy is that there is an enemy who has to be attacked or from whom it is necessary to flee. Basic assumption of pairing: there is an unconscious collective belief that, whatever the present problems and needs of the group may be, they will be solved by a future event: the birth of a child not yet conceived who will be the saviour of the group. Associated Notions: Function-experience and function-institution. Essential Bibliography: Bion, W.R. (1961) *Experiences in Groups.* Karnac Books London, 1968.

Belonging: An individual's belonging to a group, at a primitive level, depends on the fact that he has placed in the group some strongly undifferentiated and hard to represent aspects of himself (see Correale 1992). Belonging corresponds also, more realistically, to the fact that the individual acquires confidence in his right to exist within the group, and is convinced that the behaviour of the other members will confirm this right (see Goodall, 1991; S. Scheidlinger 1964). Associated Notions: Animation, Genius loci. Essential Bibliography: Lewin, K. (1948) *Resolving Social Conflicts.* Harper and Row, New York.

Bi-Personal Unconscious Phantasy (M. and W. Baranger): Bi-personal unconscious phantasy constitutes the innermost structure of the 'bi-personal field' and consists of a precipitate of the interplay of mutual projective identifications which involves to a varying extent both the patient and the analyst. Associated Notions: Field, Emotional-phantasy constellation, Essential Bibliography: Baranger, M. and Baranger, W. (1961–62). 'La situación analitica como campo dinámico.' *Revista Uraguaya de Psicoanalisis 4,* 1, 3–54.

Boundaries of the Group: The group tends to locate itself within an area of belonging which is more or less clearly defined and delimited with respect to the outside of an imaginary boundary; the boundary of the group. Associated Notions: Inside and outside, Dyadic membrane, Common space of the group. Essential Bibliography: Koyré, A. (1948) 'Du monde de l' "à-peu-près" l'univers de la précision.' In *Etudes d'histoire de la pensée philosophique.* Armand Collin, Paris.

Cannibalistic Meal (S. Freud): In a famous passage Freud describes the killing of the father-leader of the Horde and the cannibal banquet, which starts off the process which will lead to the birth of the Community of brothers, through a complex series of passages including the incorporation of the slain father, the emergence of guilt, the institution of prohibitions, the deification of the father. Freud tells us how one day the sons together took the upper hand, and after killing their father, who was at the same time their ideal enemy, ate his mortal remains together. After this criminal act none of them could take on the paternal heritage, since each of them stopped the others from doing so. From sudden loss and remorse for the crime committed the sons learned to bear with each other and unite in a fraternal clan born of the prescriptions of totemism, which guaranteed that this would never happen again; they agreed to give up possession of women, because they had killed the father on their account. They could now marry only women outside the clan. This is the origin of exogamy and its intimate connection

Character Armour (W. Reich): The poor functioning of 'mental skin' may lead a baby to form a substitute (muscular) prosthesis, to replace normal dependence on the containing object with a pseudo-independence. These phenomena have been partly described in different terminology by W. Reich (1933) who speaks of the 'muscular armour of the character'. Associated Notions: Adhesive identification, Ego-skin, Mental skin. Essential Bibliography: Reich, W. (1933) *Character Analysis*. Vision, London, 1950.

Cohesion (I. D. Yalom): According to Yalom cohesion represents one of the group's principal therapeutic factors. He defines it generically as the end result of the work of forces which operate in order to keep each member within the group or as the attraction that a group exerts on its components. Yalom also specifies that cohesion is not synonymous with acceptance and understanding. Associated Notions: Fusion, Interdependence, Solidarity. Essential Bibliography: Yalom, I.D. (1985) *The Theory and Practice of Group Psychotherapy* (3rd edition). Basic Books, New York.

Collective Unconscious (C.G. Jung): 'Images, ideas, formulations and laws are somehow stored in a social structure...'According to Jung, in socially determined memory, these elements play exactly the same role as that assigned by the traditional theory of memory to the "traces" left by individual experiences' (Bartlett 1932). Associated Notions: Historical field and actual field, Group phantasy. Essential Bibliography: Jung, C.G. (1928) *Relations between the Ego and the Unconscious. Collected Works*, Vol. 5. Routledge, London.

Commuting: With reference to group analysis, this term denotes the to and fro motion between the individual and the group dimensions. An intentional and particularly creative way of commuting is 'effective narration'. A second, non-intentional and unconscious, way of commuting, is 'trans-personal propagation'. Associated Notions: Configuration, Trans-personal diffusion, Explicitation, Effective narration. Essential Bibliography: Corrao, F. (1954) 'Duale Gruppale.' In G. Di Chiara and C. Neri (eds.) *Psicoanalisi Futura*. Borla, Rome.

Condensation (S.H. Foulkes): One of the group's functional mechanisms described by Foulkes is condensation. He attributes to the term a different meaning from the one which Freud gives it. To be more precise, Foulkes says: 'It almost seems that the collective unconscious operates as a condenser which first stores in secret the strong emotional charges generated by the group, then discharges them in the form of typical shared group events' (Foulkes and Anthony 1957, p.151) Associated Notions: Historical field and actual field, Model scene. Essential Bibliography: Foulkes, S.H. and Anthony, E.J. (1957) *Group Psychotherapy: The Psychoanalytic Approach*. Heinemann, London. Reprinted, Karnac Books, London, 1984.

Configuration (S.H. Foulkes): Foulkes and Anthony (1957, p.237) describe the notion as follows: 'Every single event in the group, even if it seems to involve only one or two members, has a certain configuration which involves the group as a whole.' Associated Notions: Commuting. Essential Bibliography: Foulkes, S.H. and Anthony, E.J. (1957) *Group Psychotherapy: The Psychoanalytical Approach*. Karnac Books, London 1989.

Container and Contained (W.R. Bion): See Glossary entry *Interaction between – and –*.

Crowd (G. Le Bon): According to Le Bon (1895), individuals when they are in a crowd, behaving according to the impulses of the crowd, independently of their life-style, their occupations, their temperament or intelligence, acquire a sort of collective mind simply because they have transformed into a crowd. This collective mind makes them feel, think, act in a completely different way from the one in which each of them would feel, think and act as an isolated individual. The psychological crowd, according to Le Bon, is a temporary thing composed of heterogeneous elements joined together for an instant. Associated Notions: Group soul, Mass.

heterogeneous elements joined together for an instant. Associated Notions: Group soul, Mass. Essential Bibliography: Le Bon, G. (1895) *The Crowd. A Study of the Popular Mind.* Fisher Unwin, London, 1921.

De-Individualisation: 'De-individualisation' is a transitory, reversible and modulated form of 'de-personalisation' which appears in the small analytic group as an aspect of the phenomenology of the 'Emerging state of the group'. It involves the disassembly of individual functioning patterns and the movement of the participants towards forms of group functioning. Associated Notions: De-personalisation, Disassembly, Emerging state of the group. Essential Bibliography: Turquet, P. (1975) 'Threats to identity in large groups.' In L. Kreeger (ed.) *The Large Group: Dynamics and Therapy.* Karnac Books, London, 1994.

De-Personalisation, Sensations of Unreality: De-personalisation and sensations of unreality occur 'physiologically' when an individual makes his first contact with a group (see Gaburri 1986a, p.111). Sometimes these phenomena are very intense, affect all the participants and have a paralysing effect on the whole group. Those present are caught up in a totalising and confusing situation, with consequent diminishing or loss of their identity. In this case the picture is very similar to one described by Bion, when he speaks of a group dominated by basic assumptions. Associated Notions: Basic assumptions, De-individualisation, Mass. Essential Bibliography: Tagliacozzo, R. (1976) 'La depersonalizzazione: crisi di rappresentazione del S, nella realtà esterna.' *Rivista di psicoanalisi 22,* 3.

Disassembly (D. Meltzer): D. Meltzer speaks of disassembly as a passive process in which the Ego and the object lose their constituting fragments because the lack of attention to themselves, to their own experiences and ways of functioning, does not allow them to set up a hierarchy of sensorial perceptions. Associated Notions: De-individualisation. Essential Bibliography: Meltzer, D. (1992) *The Claustrum. An Investigation of Claustrophobic Phenomena.* The Clunie Press, Perthshire, 1992.

Effective Narration: The 'language of effectiveness' is one of a person or group that does not judge, but is fascinated by a reality whose various evolutionary potentialities are kept open. It is the language of those who do not limit themselves to a description, but interact with whatever they are speaking about. The 'language of effectiveness' often takes the form of an 'effective narration', which is capable of putting the listener in relation with the thoughts, emotions and feelings present in the group field. Associated Notions: Commuting. Essential Bibliography: Corrao, F. and Neri, C. (1981) 'Introduction.' In C. Neri and P. Bion Talamo (eds) 'Single subject number devoted to W.R. Bion.' *Rivista di Psicoanalisi 27,* 3–4.

Egocentrism (J. Piaget): Piaget uses the term 'egocentrism' to designate the small baby's inability to recognise that different points of view can exist. According to Piaget, this inability is closely linked with the fact that the baby is not yet fully aware that he himself exists as someone different from the rest of the world. Even though egocentrism gradually dwindles, we still find it in children at nursery school and even in the juniors. Even adults are sometimes 'egocentric' and may, for example assert: 'Anyone who sees this in a different way is influenced by prejudices' (see Camaioni 1980, pp.84–93; Murphy 1951, p.479) Associated Notions: Identity as a multiple. Essential Bibliography: Piaget, J. (1926) *The Child's Representation of the World.* Kegan Paul, London, 1929.

Emerging State of the Group: The term 'emerging state' has been used by many researchers in contexts and meanings different from those given to it in this book. In particular, J. Moreno who, in his studies on creativity, uses this term to bring out the importance of spontaneity in the moment of creativity. Members of the small analytic group experience the phenomena of the 'Emerging state of the group' in an ambivalent way. Among the pleasant and positive experiences is the diffusion of feelings of expectation and hope. Among those which are burdened with anxiety, are depersonalisation and a sense of unreality. The 'Emerging state of the group' is a transitory condition which opens the way to more stable and structured attitudes in the group, such as those which characterise the 'Fraternal Community stage'. Associated Notions: Waiting for the Messiah, De-individualisation, De-personalisation, Group illusion, Homeric psychology, Primitive stage. Essential Bibliography: Neri, C. (1979b) 'La Torre di Babele: lingua, appartenenza, spazio-tempo nello stato gruppale nascente.' *Gruppo e Funzione Analitica 1*, 2–3.

Emotive-Phantasmatic Constellation: An emotive-phantasmatic constellation is a combination of emotions and phantasies, generated by the evolution of 'O', which in its turn influences group discourse and communication. An essential role in the constitution of a given emotive-phantasmatic constellation is played by the choice of the analyst and the group members, who concentrate their interest on a certain set of elements (expectations, fears, emotions, sentiments, phantasies, thoughts) from among many others which remain in the background. Associated Notions: Chosen fact, 'O', Synchronicity. Essential Bibliography: Bion, W.R. (1977) 'Catastrophic change.' *Bulletin of the British Psycho-Analytic Society 5*.

Evolution In 'O' (W.R. Bion): See note p.104. Associated Notions: Mimesis, 'O'. Essential Bibliography: Bion, W.R. (1970) *Attention and Interpretation.* Karnac Books, London, 1988; Jannuzzi, G. (1979) 'Scena primaria, contratto e scena escatologica nel "qui ed ora" del gruppo analitico.' *Gruppo e Funzione Analitica 1*, 1.

Experience-Function and Institution-Function: Experience function and institution-function come face-to-face in the life of a small group. The first occurs in the structure of the group as a small community. The second corresponds to experiencing, in the sense of Bion's 'learning from experience'. Associated Notions: Learning from experience, Work-group, Primitive mentality. Essential Bibliography: Gluckman, M. (1965) *Politics, Law and Ritual in Tribal Society.* The New American Library, New York.

Explicitation (W.R. Bion): 'The term explicitation simply means the whole of those operations necessary to transform into public knowledge the private and exclusive knowledge of the individual. The problems which it involves are of two types: technical and emotive. Emotive problems depend on the fact that man is a political animal, and is therefore prevented from showing initiative outside a group and obliged to associate the satisfaction of his own emotive tendencies with their social aspects. But given that his impulses, and not only the sexual ones, are also narcissistic, the problems connected with explicitation exist essentially in terms of conflict between narcissism and social trends. As far as technical problems are concerned, they concern the expression, through language or other signs, of thoughts or notions' (Bion 1962a, pp.180–181) Associated Notions: Commuting. Essential Bibliography: Bion, W.R. (1967) *Second Thoughts: Selected Papers on Psycho-Analysis.* Karnac Books, London, 1987.

Feedback: See note p.70. Associated Notions: Self-representation. Essential Bibliography: Bateson, G. (1972) *Steps to an Ecology of Mind.* Chandler Press, San Francisco.

Field: Initially in group psychology attempts were made to describe group phenomena and functioning through concepts exclusively concerning individuals and their reciprocal identifications, attractions and repulsions. The concept of field was at first only an instrument intended to facilitate the description of phenomena, the explanation of which, however, still remained linked to hypotheses regarding individuals. However, it became necessary to realise that in the new language the essential is the description of the field interposed between persons and not the persons themselves and their impulses. A new concept was created which had no place in the previous scheme. Slowly and not without a struggle, the concept of field ended up occupying a dominant position. For a group psychotherapist the field is now as real as the chair he is sitting on (see Einstein and Infeld 1938, p.161). Associated Notions: Semiosphere, The situaciòn analitica como campo din mico.' *Revista Uruguaya de Psicoanalisis* 4, 1, 3–54; Pichon-Riviére (1977) *El proceso gruppal. Del psicoanalisis a la psicologia social.* Nueva Visión, Buenos Aires.

Focal Conflict (D.S. Whitaker and M.A. Liebermann): 'Focal conflict' includes a 'disturbing motive' (for example, every patient's desire to have the therapist to himself); this gives rise to a 'reactive motive' (fear of the disapproval of the therapist and of the other members of the group); the result is a 'group solution' (creation of a climate of false collaboration). It is appropriate to say that Whitaker and Liebermann do not consider the 'group solution' a stable defence. The 'group solution' may change, even in the course of a single session. Associated Notions: Common tension of the group, Transference of the group. Essential Bibliography: Whitaker, D.S. and Liebermann, M.A. (1964) *Psychotherapy through the Group Process.* Atherton Press, New York.

Fraternal Community: The Fraternal Community (or fraternal clan) has various functions. Among these is the function of supporting the analyst in regulating possession of a common 'affective heritage'; in symbolic terms, in regulating the possession of women. This function is part of a triangular relationship (analyst, Fraternal Community, the group's affective heritage) which is based on a 'nomos' or fundamental right, which is not a part of the setting rules and is not present at the beginning of therapy, but which comes into being at the moment when the members become conscious of being a group (Fraternal Community stage) and begin to operate as such, becoming a 'collective subject' (see Gear and Liendo 1979). Associated Notions: The group as a collective subject, Nomos, The group's affective heritage, The Fraternal Community Stage. Essential Bibliography: Freud, S. (1912–13) *Totem and Taboo.* SE XIII.

Fraternal Community Stage: The name 'Community of brothers' was coined by Freud to indicate the phase of the mental life of the group which follows the murder of the father-leader who ruled uncontested over the primitive horde. I use Fraternal Community stage to indicate that phase of group life in which the members become a 'collective subject' capable of thought, becoming responsible for what happens in the group. Associated Notions: Fraternal Community, Group as collective subject, Work-group, Cannibalistic meal, Stage of discrimination. Essential Bibliography: Freud, S. (1921) *Group Psychology and the Analysis of the Ego.* SE XVIII.

Free Association: A method which consists of expressing without discrimination all the thoughts which come to mind, either following a given element (word, number, image of a dream, any representation), or spontaneously. The rule of free association aspires to eliminate the voluntary selection of thoughts, so that a determined order of the unconscious is brought to light. Associated Notions: Group associative chain. Essential Bibliography: Laplanche, J. and Pontalis, J.B. (1967) *The Language of Psychoanalysis.* Hogarth Press, London.

Function: The term 'function' is used in this book with two meanings, which refer respectively to the world of mathematics and to that of physiology. A function is a function, but it is also something which has a function. In so far as it is a function it has factors (for example, the capacity to tolerate frustration, the presence of a favourable environment); in so far as it has a function it also has aims (for example, it enables us to distinguish dream from waking, it frees us from an excessive accumulation of undigested emotions). Associated Notions: Function-experience and function-institution, α Function, γ Function, Genius loci. Essential Bibliography: Corrao, F. (1981) 'Struttura poliadica e funzione gamma.' *Gruppo e Funzione Analitica 2,* 2.

α-Function (W.R. Bion): See note p.45. Associated Notions: Working through. Essential Bibliography: Bion, W.R. (1992) *Cogitations.* Karnac Books, London.

γ-Function (F. Corrao): Corrao (1981, pp.30–31) suggests the name of γ- function for the element corresponding in the group to the function in the individual. The γ- function operates on the sensorial and emotive elements, generating elements available: (1) for the formation of group thoughts regarding dreams and myths etc.; (2) to differentiate the conscious from the unconscious. It is important to make clear that according to Corrao the activation of function γ implies a partial and reversible destructurisation of the α-function of the individuals who are taking part in the group. Associated Notions: α Function, Group thought. Essential Bibliography: Corrao, F. (1981) 'Struttura politica e funzione gamma.' *Gruppo e Funzione Analitica 2*, 2.

Genius Loci: In the small analytic group the 'Genius loci' refers to the function of reanimating group identity and linking the change with the affective basis of the group. Associated Notions: Belonging, Cohesion, Limits of the group, Affective heritage of the group, Syncretic sociality. Essential Bibliography: Neri, C. (1993) 'Genius loci: una funzione del luogo analoga a quella di una divinita tutelare.' *Koinos 14*, 1–2.

Group: The use of the word 'group' to indicate a 'whole' of elements is recent. In about the mid-eighteenth century the word came to be used, not only for a set of things but also for a gathering of people. The first and oldest meaning of the word was 'knot'. The sense of knot has remained within the present use of the word, indicating the cohesion of the group. The term has also been said to descend from the German *Kruppa*, that is to say, a rounded mass (see Anzieu and Martin 1968–86). Associated Notions: Coinonia. Essential Bibliography: Lo Verso, G. and Vinci, S. (1990) *Il gruppo nel lavoro clinico: bibliografia ragionata*. Giuffr, Milan; Pauletta, G. (ed) (1989) *Modelli psicoanalitici nel gruppo*. Cortina, Milan; Vanni, F. (1984) *Modelli mentali di gruppo*. Cortina, Milan.

Group Analysis: See note p.33. Associated Notions: Group analytic psychotherapy. Essential Bibliography: Slavson, S. (1964) *A Textbook in Analytic Group Psychotherapy*. International University Press, New York; Wolf, A. and Schwartz, E.K. (1970) *Beyond the Couch*. Science House, New York.

Group Analytic Psychotherapy: S.H. Foulkes (1964, p.43) suggests a precise location for 'group analytic psychotherapy', situating it both with respect to psychoanalysis and with respect to other group therapies. Foulkes says the use of the term 'Group analytic psychotherapy' stresses two aspects: first of all that in its general theoretical and clinical orientation it is situated in a common territory with psychoanalysis; and second, that because of its intensity and its aims, on the level of group therapy, it occupies a position very similar to that seen in psychoanalytical psychotherapy. Therefore, it is a psychoanalytic psychotherapy which is carried out within a group, considered as a unit. However, like other forms of psychotherapy, it also puts the single individual at the centre of attention. Associated Notions: Group analysis. Essential Bibliography: Foulkes, S.H. (1964) *Therapeutic Group Analysis*. Karnac Books, London.

Group As Collective Subject: Group thought is based on the existence of a collective subject. In its turn this depends on the fact that there is a certain continuity in the group and that solidarity has developed among the members. Associated Notions: Fraternal Community, Group thought, Solidarity. Essential Bibliography: Boas, F. (1911) *The Mind of Primitive Man*. The McMillan Company, New York.

Group As Self-Object: The Self-object is a function within the individual which is developed and maintained through constant relationship with an object of the external world which has the capacity to 'feed' it. The object in the external world which feeds the 'Self-object function' may be a group, and not only a person. Associated Notions: Affective heritage of the group. Essential Bibliography: Kohut, H. (1984) *How does Analysis Cure?* Chicago University Press, Chicago; Wolf, E.S. (1988) *Treating the Self*. Guilford Press, New York.

Group Associative Chain (R. Kaës): See panel p.35. Associated Notions: Free Associations, Resonance. Essential Bibliography: Kaës, R. (1993) *Le groupe et le sujet du groupe.* Dunod, Paris; Kaës, R. (1994) *La parole et le lien.* Dunod, Paris.

Group Atmosphere: The term indicates the background climate which immediately strikes anyone who enters a room where a group of people are gathered together. G. di Leone (1991) has suggested the word 'synaesthesia' to indicate how the multitude of things which a person perceives when taking part in a group session give way to a single comprehensive impression of the group atmosphere. For the group therapist the atmosphere is a prime source of valuable information about the possible thoughts, phantasies and moods of the group members. Associated Notions: Actual field and historical field, Trans-personal phenomena. Essential Bibliography: Redl, F. (1942) 'Group emotion and leadership.' *Psychiatry 5.*

The Group's Common Space: The 'Group's common space' is a 'functional place', cathected with affects, which is considered to be a space in which group interaction and group life take place. In the small analytic group, it gradually becomes an attractor of sensations, phantasies and thoughts. In this book the terms 'Analytic space', the 'Group's common space', 'Field' and 'Semiosphere' are for the most part interchangeable because they refer to different aspects of the same phenomenology. Associated Notions: Limits of the group, Proxemics. Essential Bibliography: Whorf, B.L. (1956) *Language, Thought and Reality.* MIT Press, Cambridge, Massachusetts.

Group Common Tension (H. Ezriel): Ezriel (1950, 1952) coined the expression 'group common tension' to describe group conflict resulting from various concomitant factors: (1) the shared relationship with the therapist which is desired yet feared (the relationship they want to avoid); (2) the phantasy relating to this relationship which arouses the fear of consequences if it were recognised (catastrophic relationship); (3) the conflict which develops in this way is resolved through the adoption of a compromise with the therapist (the required relationship). Ezriel considers that the individuation of 'group common tension' is the therapist's first task. He thinks in addition that the therapist must show every member of the group what his personal contribution to the conflict and to its solution is, on the basis of his personal pathology (see Brown and Pedder 1991, pp.122–123). Associated Notions: Focal conflict, Group transference. Essential Bibliography: Ezriel, H. (1973) 'Psychoanalytic group therapy.' In L.R. Wolberg and E.K. Schwarz, *Group Therapy: An Overview.* International Medical Books, New York.

Group Fusion (J.P. Sartre): See note p.47. Associated Notions: Fraternal Community stage. Essential Bibliography: Sartre, J.P. (1960) *Critique of Dialectical Reason.* Vols I and II. Verso Editions, London [1984 and 1991].

Group Illusion (D. Anzieu): D. Anzieu (1976) suggested the term 'group illusion' for a feeling of euphoria and great confidence in oneself and in the goodness of the experience which groups in general, and training groups in particular, experience in the early days of the group's existence. In the first works which he devoted to this theme, Anzieu considers group illusion as a defence phenomenon: the members of the group, faced with a new and difficult situation, retreat into an illusory world. In later works (1981; 1988) he reviews his position, approaching a view of illusion as a phenomenon which is partly necessary for group development. Associated Notions: Phantasy of being at one, Syncretic sociality, Emerging state of the group. Essential Bibliography: Anzieu, D. (1976) *Le groupe et l'inconscient.* Dunod, Paris; Anzieu, D. (1988) 'Introduction to D. Rosenfeld.' *Psychoanalysis and Groups,* Karnac Books, London.

Group Membrane and Dyadic Membrane: Freud describes the living organism in its most simplified form possible, as an undifferentiated bladder with a substance which can be stimulated. H. Dicks (1987) takes up Freud's idea and proposes that there are unconscious links which make the couple a unit around which there appears a kind of common Ego boundary, defined by the term 'dyadic membrane' (see Giannakoulas 1992, pp.129–130). R.D. Hinshelwood (1977) hypothesises the existence of a boundary or membrane separating the group from other groups and the various sub-groups of the same group. Associated Notions: Limits of the group, Inside and outside, Common space of the group. Essential Bibliography: Dicks, H.V. (1977) *Marital Tensions.* Routledge, London. Reprinted Karnac Books, London, 1993; Hinshelwood, R.D. (1987) *What Happens in Groups.* Free Association Books; Van Gennep, A. (1909) *Les rites de passage.* Nourry, Paris.

Group Mind: The group mind is the system of relationships which occur between the individual minds which compose it. It can also be said that the group mind is a little more and a little different from the simple sum of individual minds. It has, in fact, its own anatomical and sensorial basis, and has different functional levels. Associated Notions: Group thought, Protomental system, Super-individual thinking unit. Essential Bibliography: McDougall, M. (1927) *The Group Mind.* Cambridge, Cambridge University Press.

Group Oedipus Complex: D. Anzieu (1970, pp.352–356) writes: 'Freud's position is known: the Oedipus complex is the psychic nucleus of culture and social life…the mythical scene of the collective killing of the father would constitute the specifically group or societal version of the oedipal phantasy. My colleagues in the team and I had initially taken up this opinion without reservations…Now I am rather more critical…Here, then, is my conclusion: the Oedipus complex is the unconscious organiser of the family, it is not an organiser of the group. I am tempted to go even further; groups often use the Oedipus complex as a pseudo-organiser.' Associated Notions: Group phantasy, Group psychic organisers, Cannibalistic meal. Essential Bibliography: Freud, S. (1912–1913) *Totem and Taboo.* SE XIII. Freud, S. (1921) *Group Psychology and the Analysis of the Ego.* SE XVIII.

Group Phantasy: According to Anzieu (1976, p.359) some phantasies are active in the group in a specific way: the phantasy of the group machine is one which has to do with castration anxiety; certain silences are linked with the anxiety and phantasy of devouring; the phantasy of breaking represents a kind of common denominator of the different possible disorganisations by which the participants in a group feel threatened. Associated Notions: Emotional and phantasy constellation, Phantasm, 'O'. Essential Bibliography: Anzieu, D. (1981) *Le groupe et l'inconscient.* Dunod, Paris; Viola, M. (1981) 'Fantasma originario, fantasia e rappresentazione in un gruppo analiticamente orientato.' *Gruppo e funzione analitica 2,* 3.

Group Psychic Apparatus (R. Kaës): R. Kaës (1993, p.176) defines the group psychic apparatus as: 'the common psychic construction of the members of a group for the group. Its main characteristic is to ensure the mediation and exchange of differences between the psychic reality in its intrapsychic, intersubjective and group components, and group reality in its social and cultural aspects'. Associated Notions: Presence of the group. Essential Bibliography: Kaës, R. (1976) *L'appareil psychique groupal: Constructions du groupe.* Dunod, Paris.

Group Psychic Organisers (R. Kaës): R. Kaës (1976, p.178) distinguishes four unconscious psychic organisers of the group which are constituted from object-relations coherently articulated with the aim of instinct satisfaction: the image of the body, the original phantasy, family complexes and the image of the subjective psychic apparatus. Associated Notions: Presence of the group. Essential Bibliography: Kaës, R. (1976) *L'appareil psychique groupal: Constructions du groupe.* Dunod, Paris.

Group Soul (E. Durkheim): The hypothesis of a transpersonal matrix of psychic life was already anticipated by Durkheim (1893) in *Les regles de la methode sociologique:* 'by uniting, penetrating, relying on each other, individual souls give life to a being (psychic, if we like) which, however, constitutes a psychic individuality of a new kind. For this reason we must look into the nature of this individuality, and not that of the units which compose it, to find the reasons which have determined facts which have occurred; the group thinks, feels and acts in a quite different way from the one its members would if they were isolated. If we ignore this, we will not be able to understand anything that happens in the group'. Associated Notions: Matrix, Group mind, Super-individual units of thinking. Essential Bibliography: Durkheim, E. (1901) *Sociologie et sciences sociales. De la methode dans les sciences.* Alcan, Paris; Durkheim, E. (1897) *Suicide: A Study in Sociology.* Kegan Paul, London, 1953.

Group Thought: The term 'group mind' indicates a set of relationships. The term 'group thought' indicates a collection of operations and the product of these operations. Group thought provides self-representation for the group. It is also able to metabolise mental states burdened with anxiety which single individuals cannot work through and metabolise. It works through the 'group associative chains' and through the 'star arrangement'. One of its characteristics is the globality of the transformation with which it cathects the combination of elements which are its objects. There may be collaboration between group thought and individual thought. However, for that to happen there must be syntony (attunement) between the individual's way of thinking and the group's. Associated Notions: Self-representation, Group associative chain, Star arrangement, Group mind, γ-Function, Super-individual thinking unit. Essential Bibliography: Neri, C. (1979a) 'La culla di spago.' *Quadrangolo 4*, 1, 27–32.

Group Transference: It is as well to make a distinction between the expressions 'group transference' and 'transference in the group situation'. The first (group transference) can mean a cathexis of the whole group in the therapist or another common object. This possibility was explored by Whitaker and Liebermann (1964) who introduced the concept of 'focal conflict' and by Ezriel (1950; 1952) who speaks of 'group common tension'. The second expression, on the other hand, refers to individual transference in the group situation. Associated Notions: Group analysis, Focal conflict, Group common tension. Essential Bibliography: Rouchy, J.C. (1980) 'Processus archaiques et transfert en groupe-analyse.' *Connexions 31*; Sommaruga, P. (1981) 'Il transfert nei piccoli gruppi. Gruppo e funzione.' *Analitica 2, 3.*

Group World: The term 'group world' expresses a total and global view which could be expressed as follows: 'the group constitutes a world for the people who take part in it'. The definition 'group world' refers specifically to shared sensoriality dimensions. Phenomena connected with the 'group world' are more evident in the initial phases of the group (Emerging state of the group). Associated Notions: Group boundaries, Phantasy of being at one, Group illusion, Syncretic sociality, Emerging state of the group. Essential Bibliography: Calvino, I. (1964) 'Tutto in un punto.' In *Romanzi e racconti*, Vol. 2, Mondadori, Milan, 1992.

Homeric Psychology (W.R. Bion): This is another name Bion uses to describe the 'Primitive stage'. In fact, referring to this phase of development, Bion says that 'Homeric psychology' reigns in the group: group members imagine the Great Man as endowed with the qualities of the demigods, of the *Iliad* and the *Odyssey*, and yet as sharing common human passions such as envy, intense jealousy, rancour etc. Associated Notions: Primitive stage. Essential Bibliography: Bion, W.R. (1988) *Attention and Interpretation.* Karnac Books, London.

Idem And Autos (D. Napolitani): According to Napolitani, individuality means that part of the personality which is mostly based on imitative components. This may be confirmed by the fact that the term 'individuality' has its etymological root in *idem* and this suggests an unconscious inclination to reproduce 'interiorised scripts' in our encounters with the world. The universe of 'internal groupality', the *idem*, in the context of intrapsychic dynamism, finds its interlocutor in autos, the innovative dimension of the subject. Autos, or what is authentic, is the subjective component which can at any moment be reflected onto the 'internal groupality', and pass through it. Associated Notions: Narcissistic contract, Transpersonal diffusion, Internal groupality, Trans-psychic transmission. Essential Bibliography: Napolitani, D. (1987) *Individualità e gruppalità*, Boringhieri, Turin.

Imago: 'The concept of imago comes from Jung who describes the maternal, paternal, fraternal imago...The imago is an unconscious prototype of personages which electively directs the way in which the subject perceives others...It is not to be understood as a reflection of what is real, not even in a more or less distorted way; for example, the imago of a terrible father may very well correspond to a very gentle real father' (Laplanche and Pontalis 1967, pp.224–225). Associated Notions: Phantasm, Group phantasy. Essential Bibliography: Jung, C.G. (1912) *Symbols of Transformation: The Concept of Libido. Collected Works* Vol. 5, Routledge, London, 1956.

Immaterial Similarity (W. Benjamin): 'Immaterial similarity' is the relationship that mimesis individuates between the two terms on which it works.. Associated Notions: Mimesis. Essential Bibliography: Benjamin, W. (1919) 'Die Aufgabe des übersetzers.' In *Gesammelte Schriften*, IV–1, Suhrkamp Verlag, Frankfurt am Main, 1972; Weil, S. (1941) *Oeuvres Complètes*. Gallimard, Paris, 1991.

Induction And Abduction (C.S. Peirce): Induction and abduction have a characteristic in common: they lead one to accept a hypothesis because the facts observed are as they would necessarily or probably be as consequences of that hypothesis. The method of one, however, is exactly the opposite of the other. Induction starts with a promising hypothesis, without a particular theory in mind to begin with, although recognising the need for facts to support the theory. Abduction on the contrary starts with facts, without a particular theory in mind to begin with, although motivated by the impression that a theory is required to explain the facts. Associated Notions: Chosen fact, Synchronicity. Essential Bibliography: Bonfantini, M.A. and Grazia, R. (1976) 'Teoria del conoscenza e funzione dell'icona in Peirce.' *Versus: quaderni di studi semiotici 15*, 1; Peirce, C.S. (1878) *The Laws of Hypothesis* in C.S. Pierce (1931–1935).

Initiation: M. Meslin (1986, p.73) recalls that 'Any initiation is a complex and ambivalent phenomenon. It consists of bringing an individual, via particular instructions, to the knowledge of given things which have been hidden up till then, and introducing him into a particular group, into a secret society, in which he is called upon to live a new life. The content of this initiation can be defined as a combination of highly symbolic rites and more or less developed ethical-practical teachings, aimed at the acquisition of a certain power and wisdom based on esoteric knowledge and involving a modification of the social and religious position of the individual. In fact, after initiation, while remaining himself, this individual has become different though not really someone else, because he is still the same man, she is still the same woman, with the same physical, psychological and mental components. Initiation has simply allowed him to reach another level of existence.' M. Bernabei (1994) has established a relationship between the process of initiation and the therapeutic effectiveness of the small analytic group. Associated Notions: Animation. Essential Bibliography: Ries, J. (ed.) (1986) *Les Rites d'Initiation*. Centre d'histoire des religions, Louvain-la Neuve.

Inside and Outside: Lakoff and Johnson, in an analysis of the metaphorical structure of day-to-day language, write: 'Each of us is a container with a surface which establishes its boundaries and an inside–outside orientation. We project our inside-outside orientation on to all other physical objects which are bounded by surfaces, and we see them as containers with an inside and an outside. When we say that someone is in a room, and the room is in a house, rooms and houses are obviously containers; to move from one room to another means to move from one container to another, that is to go out of one room and into another. We attribute this orientation to solid objects, for example, when we break a piece of stone to see what is inside. Similarly we impose this orientation on our natural environment. But even when there is no natural physical boundary which could help to define a container, we impose one, dividing a territory in such a way that it has an internal part and an external surface, whether it be a wall, a hedge, a line or an abstract plane.' Associated Notions: Group boundaries, Dyadic membrane. Essential Bibliography: Lakoff, G. and Johnson, M. (1980) *Metaphors We Live By*. Chicago University Press, Chicago.

Institution (W.R. Bion): According to Bion the Institution is a function of the group corresponding to a specialised sub-group which has four basic activities: (1) to establish a distinction between the Great Man and common men (between the Ego-ideal and the Ego); (2) to contain the strong moves towards fragmentation which become active in the group every time there is real development; (3) to maintain the continuity of the group and thus watch over its tradition; (4) to collect new ideas and make them accessible to the common man (the group members) in the form of scientific laws, technical prescriptions, models of behaviour etc. (see Fadda 1984). Associated Notions: Institution function and experience function. Essential Bibliography: Kuhn, T.S. (1962) *The Structure of Scientific Revolutions*. University of Chicago Press, Chicago.

Interaction Between – and – (W.R. Bion): Bion stresses the dynamism of the interaction between container and contained: the act of containment always brings with it a transformation either of the contained or the container. An example of container–contained interaction is shown by a situation of this type: a child is crying in desperation, its mother picks it up and begins to rock it, singing: 'Here comes the big bad wolf to eat you all up ...' The child, when it was crying desperately, was prey to an uncontainable anxiety, a terror without a name. The mother held it mentally and physically in her arms, and gave the terror a shape and a name by singing the song about the wolf. The child in its turn was at once in a position to contain the anxiety, which had been transformed by the mother's containment. The container–contained model is a very general one. It can be used to describe the relationship between a mother and a child, but also between the elements present in the group field and in group thought. Associated Notions: Working through, Evolution in 'O', α-Function, γ-Function. Essential Bibliography: Nicolosi, S. (1987) 'La configurazione contenitore-contenuto.' In C. Neri *et al.* (eds) *Lettere bioniane.* Borla, Rome.

Interdependence (K. Lewin): According to Lewin (1948, p.125) the relationship between the members of the group is not based on their similarity, but on their interdependence. A group's system of interdependence is not concerned only with persons, but with all the elements of the field. Associated Notions: Synchronicity. Essential Bibliography: Lewin, K. (1948) *Resolving Social Conflicts.* Harper, New York; Lewin, K. (1951) *Field Theory in Social Science.* Harper and Row, New York; Luhmann, N. (1980) *Gesellschaftsstruktur und Semantik.* Suhrkamp Verlag, Frankfurt am Main.

Internal Groupality (D. Napolitani): By this notion Napolitani is not referring to a sort of internal 'pantheon' where significant personages in the individual's history (father, mother, etc.) are represented, but rather to the network of relational modalities in which the individual had taken part, to the representation of the relations of each individual with another and with the environment, to the meanings and the codes linked with these relations. In other words internal groupality is the result of the internalisation, by means of identifying processes, of all the relationships which the individual has been a part of right from his birth. The concept of 'internal groupality' apart from the similarity in terms, is profoundly different from the idea of 'psychic groupality' worked on by R. Kaës (1976,1993). R. Kaës developed a concept of 'psychic groupality' based on Freud's thought, that is to say the idea that the mind is structurally organised like a group. Kaes' psychic groupality notion is above all a model that suggests a representation of the structure and functionning of 1) the individual's mind 2) the psychic apparatus of the group 3) the relationship between these two. Associated Notions: Transpersonal diffusion, Idem and autos, Matrix. Essential Bibliography: Napolitani, D. (1987) Individualità e gruppalità. Boringhieri, Turin.

Internal Struggle (J. Bleger): Bleger stresses that at the origin of an internal struggle within a group, there is a wound inflicted on the 'syncretic sociality' of the whole group. The wound is often caused by too rapid a development of the group. In fact Bleger, like Bion, considers that internal divisions are manifestations of the difficulty the group experiences in proceeding towards an evolutionary transformation. Associated Notions: Genius loci, Syncretic sociality, Schism. Essential Bibliography: Bleger, J. (1970) 'El grupo como institucion y el grupo en las instituciones' in *Tenas de Psicologia.* Nueva Visiòn, Buenos Aires.

Koinonia (P. Fornari): Fornari (1987, p.137) gives the following definition: 'The group is a psychic reality which is born of the experience of space-time sharing (koinonia) of individuals communicating among themselves with the prospective of a large variety of realistic or imaginary, self-centred or hetero-centred goals.' Associated Notions: Group, The group's common space. Essential Bibliography: Trentini *et al.* (1987) *Il Cerchio Magico.* Angeli, Milan.

Learning From Experience (W.R. Bion): Learning from experience is a discipline capable of radically modifying the personality of the individual and the structure of the group which practises it. Learning by experience is one of the elements on which the work-group's mentality is based. Bion, in *Experiences in Groups* (1961, p.107), specifies: 'An integral part [of the work-group] is not only the idea of '"development" instead of "being endowed by instinct", but also the awareness of the value of a rational or scientific approach to the problem. An indispensable corollary of the idea of development is that the group accepts the validity of learning from experience'. Associated Notions: Function-experience and Function-institution. Essential Bibliography: Bion, W.R. (1962b) *Learning from Experience.* London, Karnac Books, 1991.

Localisation of a Disturbance (S.H. Foulkes): If we consider a psychological disturbance as mainly localised in the interaction between persons, it follows that it can never be totally attributed to a single person. For example, in the course of analytic work it may emerge that the most important cause of the disturbance is not in the patient at all, but perhaps in his wife, father-in-law etc. It is appropriate to add that if we are talking from the point of view of a 'network' and 'matrix', the emphasis moves to causes of disturbance which are different from those given in a genetic explanation which considers those dating back to childhood (see Foulkes 1948, pp.47 and 131) Associated Notions: Commuting. Essential Bibliography: Foulkes, S.H. (1948) *Introduction to Group-Analytic Psychotherapy.* Karnac Books, London, 1991.

Mass: The term 'mass' is used in this book either to refer to a multitude (a very large number of people) or to indicate a psychological condition ('mass' in the sense defined by Freud in 1921). The 'psychological condition of mass' is often met with in large assemblies (sociological mass) but may also be found in groups such as analytic groups with a small number of participants (see Russo 1993, pp.65–70). In the phase of 'Emerging state of the group' conditions appear which are similar to those of the mass group. However, they are transitory phenomena which are rapidly resolved, and then group thought begins. Associated Notions: Anomia, De-personalisation and sense of unreality, Artificial masses, Totalitarian masses, Primitive mentality, Seriality, Emerging state of the group. Essential Bibliography: Canetti, E. (1960) *Masse und Macht.* Claassen Verlag, Hamburg.

Matrix (S.H. Foulkes): Foulkes' use of the term 'matrix' instead of 'mother' is significant. A mother is someone who has given birth to a person. The matrix is the common ground from which a group or a multitude has been generated. According to Foulkes, the matrix is also the common element which allows communication between the members of a group. 'The group represents a social situation in which the patients enter into inter-reactive contact with each other: the dynamics of the group work within a common interpersonal matrix' (Foulkes 1964, p.104). Associated Notions: Medium, Network. Essential Bibliography: Foulkes, S.H. (1964) *Therapeutic Group Analysis.* Karnac Books, London.

Medium (M. McLuhan): Psychological studies, based on the information theory and before McLuhan, were more concerned with the analysis of contents than of the medium: what was considered important in communication was the message, independently of the medium used to transmit it. McLuhan on the other hand put the accent on the media of communication, seeking to get to know the characteristics of each medium and evaluating their effect on communication and on comprehension of the messages (see Fischer 1987). Associated Notions: Trans-personal phenomena. Essential Bibliography: McLuhan, M. (1977) *From the Eye to the Ear.* Harcourt Brace Jovanovitch, New York.

Meeting Group: '"Meeting group" is a fairly rough and imprecise name which covers a variety of forms. Suffice it to consider its synonyms: human relations group, T-group, marathon group, human potential group, sensorial awareness group, basic meeting group, truth-laboratory, experience group, confrontation group and so on...The participants [in the meeting group] are generally not labelled as patients; the experience is not considered as a therapy, but a growth' (Yalom 1985, p.489). Associated Notions: T-group. Essential Bibliography: Badolato, G. and Di Iullo, M.G. (1978) *Gruppi terapeutici e gruppi di formazione.* Bulzoni, Rome; Rogers, C. (1970) *Carl Rogers on Encounter Groups.* Harper, New York.

Mental Skin (E. Bick): 'The English psychoanalyst Esther Bick has perfected the methodology of systematic observation of small babies, and she has shown that, in their most primitive, psyche parts are not yet differentiated from the body parts and are seen as being deprived of that binding force which can ensure a link for them. They have to be held together in a passive form thanks to the skin which functions as a peripheral boundary. The internal function of containing the parts of the Self results from the interjection of an external object capable of containing the parts of the body. This containing object is normally constituted in the course of feeding, thanks to the dual experience which the baby has of the mother's nipple held in its mouth and its own skin held by the skin of its mother cradling it, by her warmth, by her voice, by her familiar smell. The containing object is experienced concretely as a skin' (Anzieu 1985, p.236). Associated Notions: Adhesive identification, Ego-skin. Essential Bibliography: Bick, E. (1968) *The Experience of the Skin in Early Object-relations.* Tavistock Publications, London.

Mimesis (W. Benjamin): According to Benjamin the term 'mimesis' indicates the capacity to represent something and at the same time to make it seem emotionally and almost sensorially present. Sometimes what is actualised in the small analytic group through mimetic imitation (mimesis) is not something contained in the group but a profound experience of one of the participants. Associated Notions: Evolution in 'O', Immaterial similarity. Essential Bibliography: Benjamin, W. (1933) 'Über das mimetische Vermögen.' In *Gesammelte Schriften*, II–1. Suhrkamp Verlag, Frankfurt am Main, 1977.

Mystic (W.R. Bion): According to Bion, after the group has made a distinction between man and divinity, an outstanding individual (the Mystic) aspires to re-establish direct contact with the divinity from whom he is conscious of having been separated, without the mediation of the Institution. His activity in the group is constantly directed at trying to form an intersection with the divinity and with the new idea which originated the group. Because of his efforts and his activity, this individual becomes a new hero for the group. In effect, the Mystic, who tries to establish direct contact with the divinity (with the lost Hero) is seen as a new incarnation of the Hero. His evolutionary and destructive impact corresponds to a new cycle: activation of primitive stage phenomena, the movement from the primitive stage to the stage of discrimination etc. This new cycle will bring further expansion of group reality with respect to the boundaries reached through the intuitions of previous 'outstanding individuals' and to the view of the world which the Institution has systematised on the basis of their intuitions (see Brutti and Parlani 1983, pp.51–53). Associated Notions: Institution, Stage of discrimination, Primitive stage. Essential Bibliography: Bion, W.R. (1970) *Attention and Interpretation.* London, Karnac Books, 1988.

Model Of Action (J.D. Lichtenberg): Lichtenberg attributes to the newborn baby a predisposition to interact with the mother, which is important from the point of view of the development of its capacities. In particular, he has studied the association of a certain set of sensations and experiences and a given interactive sequence. When a certain set of physical sensations and experiences is repeatedly associated with a certain interactive sequence, we can speak of the experience's 'model of action'. To give an example: a baby is hungry and sends signals for the mother to feed it; the mother responds by offering it her breast, speaking softly and smiling; the baby sucks her nipple, puts its hands on her breast and gazes with satisfaction at the mother. Given that the physical sensations and emotional reactions of this episode are repeated several times a day and for many months, the baby experiences lactation as a 'model of action' within which it acquires a constantly increasing personal and relational competence. Associated Notions: Model scene. Essential Bibliography: Lichtenberg, J.D. (1983) *Psychoanalysis and Infant Research.* London, Karnac Books.

Model Scene (J.D. Lichtenberg): Lichtenberg states that in the analytic situation, determined experiences of the analysand are frequently expressed in a certain interactive sequence, in which he may involve the analyst. This interactive sequence, which is repeated again and again and which Lichtenberg calls 'model of action' becomes progressively better understood and acquires a greater representational significance for the analyst and the analysand. We can then speak of 'model scene'. In the couple or group analytic situation, through the 'models of action' and 'model scenes', sensations and experiences appear which are not well differentiated and which initially do not correspond to a well-defined phantasy. Associated Notions: Self-representation, Model of action. Essential Bibliography: Lichtenberg, J.D. (1992) *Self and Motivational System.* Analytic Press, Hillsdale.

Multiple Identity: The identity which builds up in the group is the result of the introjection of numerous co-existent items in a dialogue or in opposition to each other. It is also multiple because it is the effect of identification with the group as a multivocal whole. Finally, it is multiple because it is the result of continual mobile differentiations regarding one or another of the points of view present in the group. Associated Notions: Animation, Social speech. Essential Bibliography: Bakhtin, M. (1984) *Problems of Dostoevsky's Poetics,* UMP..

'O' (W.R. Bion): Bion indicates by the letter 'O' 'the unknown', 'the truth', 'the divinity which contains in itself all the as yet undeveloped distinctions'. Bion's idea of 'O' can also be likened to Kant's 'thing in itself'. 'In Kant's philosophy the thing-in-itself represents the unknowable, that which remains by definition beyond the knowledge of phenomena. This knowledge can progress, but cannot reach the very foundations of reality, the precise thing-in-itself (Dazzi 1987, pp.406–441). 'O' is not only unattainable, it is also evolutionary. In the importance given to this characteristic, Bion's position is comparable to the point of view of Charles Peirce. Peirce (1931–1935) maintains that there are not only subjects who know, but that the 'thing to know' has its own evolution towards knowledge and the subjects who know it. Associated Notions: Waiting for the Messiah, Evolution in 'O'. Essential Bibliography: Amabili, B. (1993) 'O: pensiero rappresentato da un segno, cornice di un punto espanso.' In M. Bernabei and C. Neri (eds.) 'Single theme number devoted to "the symbol" in Bion.' *Metaxù 16*, 49–53.

Oedipus: See entry *Oedipus complex in the group.*

Oedipus Complex in the Group: D. Anzieu (1976, pp.352-356) writes: 'Freud's position is well known: the Oedipus complex is the psychic nucleus of culture and social life…the mythical scene of the collective killing of the father constitutes in a specific way the group or society version of the oedipal phantasy. My colleagues and I in the team had initially taken up this position without reservations…Now I am rather more critical…Here, then is my conclusion: the Oedipus complex is the unconscious organiser of the family, it is not an organiser of the group. I am tempted to go even further; groups often use the Oedipus complex as a pseudo-organiser.' Associated Notions: Group phantasy, Group psychic organisers, Cannabalistic meal. Essential Bibliography: Freud, S. (1912–1913) *Totem and Taboo*. SE XIII; Freud, S. (1921) *Group Psychology and the Analysis of the Ego*. SE XVIII.

Oedipus Myth: See *Oedipus complex in the group*.

Open Group: 'Open groups' are particularly used as reception groups in general and psychiatric hospitals, to offer patients the chance to familiarise themselves with the structure and become a part of it. Many communities have a group meeting at a prearranged hour, which is open to all patients wishing to take part. Often these groups are led, not by one therapist, but in turn by members of the staff who are on duty at that time. Associated Notions: Slow-open groups and closed groups. Essential Bibliography: Brown, D. and Pedder, J. (1991) *Introduction to Psychotherapy* (2nd edn). Routledge, London.

Organised Group (W. Mcdougall): See note p.23. Associated Notions: Work-group, Function-experience and function-institution. Essential Bibliography: Cruciani, P. (1983) 'Sighele, Le Bon, Trotter e McDougall: Le fonte di Psicologia delle masse.' In C. Neri (ed.) *Prospettive della ricerca psicoanalitica di gruppo*. Kappa, Rome.

Original Mythical Contract: Fornari (1971) has shown how every institution and every community is built around a few basic original and highly emotionally charged phantasies. A. Missenard (1989) draws attention to the importance of the 'founders': the initiators of the group. A. Correale (1991) speaks of an 'original mythical contract', highlighting the fact that from the very beginning therapeutic groups contain within them a body of specific requirements, phantasies and affects, for example powerful individual transformation phantasies which are in some way accepted and encouraged by the therapist. These elements are also important for the building up of the 'affective heritage' of the small analytic group. Associated Notions: Nomos, Affective heritage. Essential Bibliography: Weber, M. (1988) *The Protestant Ethic and the Spirit of Capitalism*. Roxbury Publishing Co., Los Angeles.

Paranoiagenesis (E. Jaques): Jaques (1955) coined the term 'paranoiagenesis' with reference to paranoiac regressions, the possibility of which is constantly present in organisations. It is manifested when the group at a loss puts enormous pressure on the leader to become paranoiac or self-critical, aggressive or indulgent. Associated Notions: Basic assumptions, Totalitarian masses. Essential Bibliography: Jaques, E. (1955) 'Social systems as defence against persecutory and depressive anxiety.' Contribution to the psychoanalytic study of social processes. In M. Klein, P. Heimann and R. Money-Kyrle (eds) *New Directions in Psychoanalysis*. Hogarth Press, London. Reprinted, Karnac Books, London, 1977.

Phantasm: The two words in English, 'phantasm' and 'phantom' correspond to the French words 'phantasme' and 'phantome'. The term 'phantom' indicates something fairly concrete: a ghost, an apparition, a creature with flowing robes and chains. The term phantasm tends more to indicate a phantasy. In French and English psychoanalysis the 'phantasm' is not only a phantasy, but something more: it is an imaginary scenario in which the subject is present, and in which he represents, in a way which is more or less distorted by defensive processes, the realisation of an unconscious wish. Associated Notions: Group phantasy, Model scene. Essential Bibliography: Laplanche, J. and Pontalis, J.B. (1967) *The Language of Psychoanalysis.* Hogarth Press, London.

Phantasy of 'Being One': The phantasy of 'being one' may be imagined in connection with external or internal objects; it may be conscious or unconscious. It may be established not only with a mother or with a partner, but also with a group, a clan or a family. In this book I use the term 'phantasy of being one' in preference to 'fusionality', which was introduced by L. Pallier, G. Petacchi, R. Tagliacozzo and G.C. Soavi as well as myself (1990), in the context of individual psychoanalytical work. The reason for this choice is the need to avoid overlapping with the term 'fusion' used by J.P. Sartre (1960) to indicate an aspect of the process of group constitution. Associated Notions: World-group, Group illusion, Syncretic sociality. Essential Bibliography: Fachinelli, E. (1983) *Claustrofilia: saggio sull'orologio telepatico in psicoanalisi.* Feltrinelli, Milan; Neri, C. *et al.* (1990) *Fusionalità: Scritti di psicoanalisi clinica.* Borla, Rome.

Picture: The term 'picture' is used, especially by the French psychoanalysts (tableau or cadre), to describe the set of arrangements necessary for analytic work to take place. The etymology of the French word *cadre* (frame) stresses particularly the delimiting aspect of the setting. However, in a psycho-analytic context, through the thought of the group, the 'picture' regains its symbolic function, allowing the representation of the deepest experiences of the participants. The 'picture', in its archaic aspect, may be considered as a containing skin which 'keeps together' the parts of the personality, thus recalling the containing function attributed by E. Bick (1968) to the skin, and by D. Anzieu (1986) to the Ego-skin (see Petrella 1993). Associated Notions: Setting-process and Setting-institution. Essential Bibliography: Kaës, R. *et al.* (1980) *L'institution et les institutions.* Dunod, Paris.

Plexus (S.H. Foulkes): During psychotherapeutic treatment the patient tends to put in dynamic connection with his conflicts a relatively small number of people who have particular significance for the disturbance. Foulkes calls this group of people the plexus, that is to say, the dynamic network within which the illness originated, and in reality what appears in the patient is simply the symptom of a disturbance in the equilibrium of the dynamic network of which he is a part (see Longo 1983, p.91). Associated Notions: Network. Essential Bibliography: Foulkes, S.H. (1975) *Group Analytic Psychotherapy.* Karnac Books, London, 1991.

Polarisation: The term is used in this book with two different meanings. The first corresponds to Foulkes' indications and refers to how the various aspects of the same phantasmatic nucleus are expressed by the different participants in the group. The second indicates how a certain emotion or tension (for example, hate) may occupy (polarise) the whole field of the group. Associated Notions: Transtemporal diffusion, Interdependence. Essential Bibliography: Foulkes, S.H. (1964) *Therapeutic Group Analysis.* Karnac Books, London.

Presence of the Group: The 'presence of the group' is an effective fiction relating to the existence of a 'common group object' which serves to reconcile the thoughts and phantasies of the various participants, giving support to group thought. Associated Notions: Group thought. Essential Bibliography: Bion, W.R. (1963) *Elements of Psychoanalysis.* Karnac Books, London, 1989; Kaës, R. (1976) *L'appareil psychique groupal: Constructions du groupe.* Dunod, Paris.

Present Field and Historical Field (A. Correale): See panel p.62. Associated Notions: Group atmosphere, Setting process and setting institution. Essential Bibliography: Correale, A. (1991) *Il campo istituzionale.* Borla, Rome.

Primitive Mentality (W.R. Bion): According to Bion, the primitive mentality of the group is characterised by the uniformity of mental activity unique to the individuals who operate under its influence. The mechanism which leads to the formation of group mentality is described by Bion (1961, p.58) in terms of anonymous contributions. 'I put forward...the hypothesis that group mentality is a common reservoir into which everyone's contributions flow anonymously and in which the impulses and desires which these contributions contain can be gratified. Each contribution to this group mentality must contain the support of other anonymous contents of the group or conform to them.' Associated Notions: Basic assumptions, Bi-personal unconscious phantasy. Essential Bibliography: Bion, W.R. (1961) *Experiences in Groups.* Karnac Books, London, 1968.

Primitive Stage (W.R. Bion): According to Bion (1970, pp.103-104 and 159–160) during the primitive stage the distinction between the members and the one who will later be recognised as the Exceptional Individual, the Great Man, has not yet been established. Correspondingly, in the individual psyche the Ego is not well-differentiated from that which will later become the Ego-ideal. In this phase it may seem that equality reigns in the group and that there are no prohibitions. It would, however, be more exact to say that there is no ability to discriminate; there are no conflicts because the differences have not yet been perceived. Associated Notions: Homeric psychology, Emergent state of the group. Essential Bibliography: Bion, W.R. (1970) *Attention and Interpretation.* Karnac Books, London, 1988.

Private Space of the Self (M.M.R. Khan): Psychanalysis has strongly emphasised the importance for the patient of the experience of communicating his states of mind and sharing them with the analyst. In certain cases, however, it is just as important that his need 'not to communicate' and 'not to share' should be respected. M. Khan wonders whether the need to keep a private space at all costs is a form of relationship with the true Self, or whether it represents, on the contrary, a paranoid and aggressive exclusion of the others from any link with him. He concludes that experiencing a private state, one that is impossible to share, is indispensable before it is possible to succeed in relating to the others symbolically, and at the same time being aware of the communication. Considering it from this particular perspective, psycho-analysis may be defined as 'a discipline which concerns the most intimate private space of life, a discipline which demands sensitivity and ability. Its practice multiplies this private space, extending it to the very particular relationship which arises between two persons who, by the very nature of their exclusive bond, change each other reciprocally' (Khan 1974, pp.11 and 206–211). Associated Notions: Egocentrism, Totalitarian masses. Essential Bibliography: Khan, M.M.R. (1974) *The Privacy of the Self.* Hogarth Press, London. Reprinted Karnac Books, London, 1996.

Protomental System (W.R. Bion): See note p.86. Associated Notions: Trans-personal diffusion. Localisation. Matrix. Essential Bibliography: Bion, W.R. (1961) *Experiences in Groups.* Karnac Books, London, 1968.

Proxemics (E.T. Hall): Hall (1966) has defined Proxemics as the field of research which concerns space where its function is to be the means for modulating social relationships. Hall emphasises that space is cathected with an affective burden, giving rise to protective reactions in the event of intrusion. Hall was also interested in the distance between individuals, and the way this distance is determined by culture and other social and environmental psychological factors. Associated Notions: Self-representation. Essential Bibliography: Hall, E.T. (1966) *The Hidden Dimension.* Doubleday, New York.

Psychic Groupality (R. Kaës): Freud's concept of the unconscious as a split group of thoughts involves the notion of psychic groupality, arranged by original, primary and secondary processes. R. Kaës (1976) has put forward this notion to describe an intrapsychic formation equipped with linking functions between drives, object, representations and agents, the whole constituting a system of fixed or transformable relations: the identification network, the distributive, permutative and dramatic structure of primal phantasies, the agents of the psychic apparatus, the systems of object relations, complexes and images are examples of internal groups.

Internal groups are a twofold organisation: they are general structures for linking inherent in psychic life, and they are specific constructions acquired through anaclisis, identification and internalization of relation schemas. Internal groups work as psychical organisers of intersubjective linkings: thus, they are constitutive principles of the group psychic apparatus. Associated Notions: Group psychic apparatus, Group psychic organisers. Essential Bibliography: Kaës, R. (1976) *L'appareil psychique groupal*. Dunod, Paris; (1993) *Le groupe et le sujet du groupe*. Dunod, Paris.

Psychic Transmission: Freud uses four different terms for the concept of psychic transmission: (1) *die Übertragung* designates (together with other terms which have the same root), the fact of transmitting, or transmittability, psychoanalytical transference, translation, transduction and communication by contagion; (2) *die Vererbung* designates what is transmitted by heredity; (3) *die Erwerbung* designates acquisition as a result of transmission; (4) *die Erblichkeit* designates heredity. This accurate choice of terms is a testimony to the fact that he considered the process of transmission between the different generations a very complex one (see Hubermann 1994). Associated Notions: Narcissistic Contract, Transpsychic transmission. Essential Bibliography: Kaës, R. *et al.* (1993) *Transmission de la vie psychique entre generations*. Dunod, Paris.

Psychodrama: See note p.71. Associated notions: Self-representation and semiosphere. Essential Bibliography: Moreno, J. (1948) *Psychodrama*. Beacon House, New York; Moreno, J. (1954) *Who Shall Survive? Foundations of Sociometry, Group Psychotherapy and Psychodrama*. Beacon House, New York.

Resonance: See note p.34. Associated Notions: Group associative chain, α Function, Working through, mirror reaction. Essential Bibliography: Foulkes, S.H. (1964) *Therapeutic Group Analysis*. London: George Allen and Unwin.

Reverie (W.R. Bion): See under α-*Function* in the Glossary.

Schism: Bion (1961, p.169) suggests the following definition: 'The defence offered by schism against the threat of a development can be detected in the operation carried out by schismatic groups which are apparently opposed to each other, but are in fact tending towards the same end. A group often adheres to the group on which it depends as to a "bible", a sacred text of the group. This group promulgates already accepted ideas, and by stripping them of every attribute to which it would be painful to adjust, it keeps the loyalty of those who wish to avoid the anxieties which development would cause. Thought is thus evened out and becomes flat and dogmatic. On the other hand, the group that is apparently supporting the new ideas becomes so exacting in its demands that it no longer succeeds in attracting adherents. Thus both groups will avoid that painful mixture of the primitive and the rational which is at the centre of the conflict caused by development.' Associated Notions: Genius loci, Internal struggle, Syncretic sociality. Essential Bibliography: Bion, W.R. (1961) *Experiences in Groups*. Karnac Books, London, 1968.

Selected Fact (W.R. Bion): A certain collection of data may appear as a heterogeneous one unless the individuation of an image gives them a sense. An example of this type of process is Kekul's dream. Kekul had analysed a new substance and was looking for its structural formula. In the course of this research he had already written a large number of linear chains composed of that certain number of atoms of carbon, oxygen and hydrogen, which he knew, and respecting the number of values known to him. Nevertheless, Kekul, could not determine the formula. During the night he dreamed of a fire-breathing dragon biting its tail. The image reorganised the data. The following morning he wrote the first formula of the organic chemical: it was not a linear chain, but a ring, the ring of benzene (see Correale 1987, p.106). Associated Notions: Emotional-phantasy constellation, Induction and abduction. Essential Bibliography: Correale, A. (1987) 'PsD.' In C. Neri *et al.* (eds) *Lettere Bioniane*. Borla, Rome; Pomar, R. (1987) 'La congiunzione costante in W.R. Bion.' In C. Neri *et al.* (eds.) *Lettere bioniane*. Borla, Rome.

Self-Object: See *Group as Self-object* in the Glossary.

Self-Representation: Self-representation is the process through which the group produces images of itself and of what is happening within it. The process of self-representation is one of the functions which characterise the 'semiosphere' of the small analytic group. Associated Notions: Feedback, Model of action, Model scene, Semiosphere. Essential Bibliography: Corrao, F. (1992) *Modelli psicoanalitici: mito, passione, memoria.* Laterza, Rome-Bari.

Semiosphere: The 'semiosphere' is the active sensing system of the small group, and also comprises all the signs, symbols and rituals which constitute the basis and the means of communication of the group. It is important to make clear that the Semiosphere implies a part–whole effect. Every intervention of one of the members of the group, since it is located in this set of meanings and relationships, is carried out and acts, not only in the context of interpersonal relations, but in the more comprehensive one of the Semiosphere of the group. Associated Notions: Field, Social speech, Common space of the group. Essential Bibliography: Lotman, J.M. (1985) *La semiosfera, l'assimmetria e il dialogo delle strutture pensanti.* Marsilio, Venice.

Seriality (J.P. Sartre): A certain number of people waiting for a bus have the same immediate aim, are exposed to the same discomfort. Despite the existence of these common conditions, they may not be a group. Each of them may be isolated from each of the others. They may be like numbers in a series. If 'group fusion' takes place, on the other hand, a feeling of 'we' arises, and they can act as a group to modify the situation they are in. Associated Notions: Anomia, Group fusion. Essential Bibliography: Sartre, J.P. (1960) *Critique of Dialectical Reason.* London, 1976.

Setting: See *Picture* and *Setting-process and setting-institution* in the Glossary.

Setting-Process and Setting-Institution (J. Bleger): Bleger (1967a, p.235) distinguishes in the 'analytic situation', one aspect which he calls 'setting-process', from a second aspect which he calls 'setting-institution'. The setting-process is a device formed of a set of rules and procedures capable of activating the basic emotions present in the group. Another set of procedures and rules of the setting-process implies that these emotions are not acted out, but are expressed through what the participants say in the session, and the way in which they say it. A final set of procedures, which is an integral part of the setting-process, is used to separate, and then put into contact, two mental states analysis participants, with very different characteristics: the first involved in emotions, the second waiting to receive signs and signals. The setting-institution, on the contrary, includes the less dynamic elements of the analytic situation, those which are characterised by long lasting and invariant aspects such as the room, the timetable, payment, holiday plans, the analyst's role. The setting-institution is a depository for the psychotic aspects of the identity, and also for the unchanging part of Self. In its turn this unchanging part of the identity is a basis and a source of security for a more mature identity. Associated Notions: Present field and historical field, Picture, Syncretic sociality. Essential Bibliography: Bleger, J. (1966a) 'Psychoanalyse du cadre psychoanalytique.' In R. Kaës *et al. Crise, rupture et dépassement. Introduction à l'analyse transitionelle.* Dunod, Paris.

Skin-Ego (D. Anzieu): D. Anzieu (1985, pp.236–237) uses the word 'Skin-ego' to mean a representation which the baby uses during the early phases of its development, in order to represent itself as Ego containing psychic contents, starting right from its experience of the surface of the body. The Skin-ego finds its support in the different functions of the skin. The first is that of a bag which contains and keeps inside what is good and satisfying, things which feeding, caring and a stream of words have accumulated in it. The skin's second function is to be the separating surface (interface) which denotes its boundaries with the outside and keeps the outside out; it is the barrier which provides protection from the penetration by the greed and aggression of others, be these beings or objects. The third and final function of the skin is, simultaneously with the mouth, and at least as much as this is, a place and a means of primary communication with others, with whom significant relations are to be established; it is also a surface on which the traces of these relations are written. Associated Notions: Limits of the group, Mental skin. Essential Bibliography: Anzieu, D. (1985) *Le moi-peau.* Bordas, Paris.

Slow-Open Group, Closed Group: Most groups composed of out-patients are slow-open groups, in which the participants change as some people leave the group when appropriate, and are replaced by others. Other groups are closed groups: all the patients begin and end together after a certain prearranged time. Closed groups are more frequent when intended for training. The prearranged ending, in fact, enables the limits imposed, for example the end of the university year, to be better respected. Associated Notions: Open group. Essential Bibliography: Brown, D. and Pedder, J. (1979) *Introduction to Psychotherapy.* Routledge, London 1991.

Social Speech (M. Bakhtin): Homer made the heroes of the *Iliad* and the *Odyssey* exclaim: 'What has come from the cloister of my teeth!!?' Something similar could have been said by the members of a small analytic group. In the small group, every word, as soon as it is pronounced, is subjected to tensions, interpretations and transformations which are the effect of the thought and speech of other participants. The sense of a dream, for example, at the moment at which a member tells it, has not only a personal significance, but is also, and above all, what emerges from the speech and transformation to which it is subjected. The analytic group is a multidiscursive and multivocal situation. Every word and every thought conceives its own object through the mist (or, on the contrary, through the light) of the words and thought of others. Associated Notions: Multiple identity, Group thought. Essential Bibliography: Bakhtin, M. (1981) 'Forms of time and of chronotope in the novel'. In *The Dialogic Imagination: Four Essays by M.M. Bakhtin.* University of Texas Press, Austin.

Solidarity (E. Durkheim): Durkheim distinguishes two forms of solidarity: mechanic and organic. The first derives from the indifferentiation of the individual; the second is linked to the need for everyone to fulfil a function which is indispensable in its own way. Associated Notions: Interdependence, Valency. Essential Bibliography: Durkheim, E. (1897) *Suicide: A Study in Sociology.* Kegan Paul, London, 1952.

Specular Reaction (S.H. Foulkes): The individual members of the small analytic group see themselves or part of themselves – often a repressed part – reflected in the interactions of the other members. This reflection helps them to know themselves through the reactions of others or the image of themselves which others show them. It is important to clarify that Foulkes emphasises that 'mirroring phenomena' refer to the group considered as a whole even when they seem to involve only one or a few participants. It is also necessary to distinguish the 'specular reactions' described by Foulkes from both the 'mirror phase' described by Lacan (1949) and the 'mirroring self object' to which H. Kohut (1984) has drawn attention. Associated Notions: Group associative chain, α-Function, Resonance. Essential Bibliography: Foulkes, S.H. (1948) *Group Analytic Psychotherapy.* Karnac Books, London, 1991.

Star Arrangement: Characteristic of the 'star arrangement' is the fact that the interests of the members of the group revolve around a common object. The argument takes place from different points of view (syncrises) by the overlapping of images relating to the same theme (thematic amplification). The result of these operations is to bring to light a present, but implicit, significance which otherwise would have difficulty in emerging because it is not based on a background sufficient to enable it to be perceived. Associated Notions: Evolution in 'O', Mimesis. Essential Bibliography: Perelman, C. and Olbrechts-Tyteca, L. (1958) *Trait, de l'argumentation.' La nouvelle rhetorique.* Paris: PUF.

Super-Individual Thinking Unit: The expression 'Super-individual thinking unit' refers either to super-organisms (like bee colonies), or to groups of people. 'Thinking units of a higher order' are distinguished from inferior ones by the fact that the individual taking part does not lose the personal exercise of his own thought. The advantage of this order of 'thinking unit' is the ductility of thought, the disadvantage is that information is not passed automatically from the group to individuals; consequently communication must be continuously sought out and adjusted. Associated Notions: Attunement, Group mind, Protomental system. Essential Bibliography: Lotman, J.M. (1993) 'La cultura e l'esplosione: prevedibilità e imprevedibilità Feltrinelli, Milan.

Syncretic Sociality (J. Bleger): One aspect of 'syncretic sociality' is to be together without the need of words. Isabel Allende in *The House of the Spirit* tells of Clara, a child (later a woman and the wife of senator Duarte) who periodically stopped speaking. This happened for the first time during her childhood. Clara stopped speaking after the death of her sister, for which she felt guilty because of her paranormal powers. The second time it happened was during her marriage: Clara was in continual political and ideological conflict with her husband, whom she loved tenderly and passionately. Her husband, Senator Duarte, after a very painful separation from Clara, suggested: 'I do not want you to speak to me, but I should be pleased to be wherever you are.' And this is what they did. Avoiding speech (she and the senator communicated only indirectly, through a third person) they succeeded for a certain time in maintaining a level of relationship (the syncretic one of being together in the same house and in the same room). But Senator Duarte and Clara's attempt failed. Syncretic society, in fact, cannot be kept separate in a stable way from 'evolved sociality'. Associated Notions: Phantasy of 'being one', Genius loci, Group world, Internal struggle. Essential Bibliography: Bleger, J. (1967b) *Simbiosis y ambigüedad.* Paidós, Buenos Aires.

Synchronicity (C.J. Jung): Jung asserted that if a certain series of events, even if they are apparently dissimilar, has taken place in a given unit of time, for example in the same session of analysis, through the principle of synchronicity, then their coincidence must be considered significant. The optics of synchronicity are found to be valuable when we have a theoretical and technical approach to the group which values the idea of the field. In fact thinking in terms of synchronicity allows us to think of facts, phantasies and thoughts told by various members of the group as being linked together by significance even if they refer to places and times which are different and distant from each other. Associated Notions: Field, Emotional and phantasmatic constellation, Chosen fact, Inference and abduction, Interdependence, Time. Essential Bibliography: Jung, C.G. (1948) 'Preface to the anonymous I Ching.' *Collected Works* Vol. 11. Routledge, London, 1958.

T-Group: The T-group is a form of training group, usually a residential one. As far as possible, the group is made up of people who do not know each other. It meets for a minimum of 5 days and a maximum of 15. The 'small group' sessions may last from an hour and a half to three hours and there may be 'plenary sessions' from time to time. Three or four sessions can take place in one day. The sessions may be alternated with exercises and seminars aimed at providing information and rationalising experience. It is made clear that the leader's task is to facilitate observation, reflection and analysis of whatever happens in the course of interaction (see Vender 1992). Associated Notions: Meeting group. Essential Bibliography: Yalom, I.D. (1985) *Theory and Practice of Group Psychotherapy* (4th edn). Basic Books, New York.

Time: Languages like French and Italian have only one word (*temps, tempo*), where there are two in English (weather, time) and German (*Wetter, Zeit*). Weather is meteorological, time is what we see on the clock. English and German are more precise than the Romance languages. However the connection between chronological time and meteorological weather may also be considered as an enrichment. The Romance conception of time shows a link between a succession of events and that space-time in which complex transformations occur relating to a multiplicity of facts which are linked and interdependent in various ways. Associated Notions: Interdependence,

Synchronicity. Essential Bibliography: Marramao, G. (1992) Kairòs. *Apologia de tempo debito.* Laterza, Rome-Bari.

Totalitarian Masses: Totalitarian masses are a particular type of artificial mass in which the individual as a centre of autonomous thoughts and emotions is systematically and actively attacked and the integrity of his 'Private space of Self' is assailed. Associated Notions: Mass, Artificial masses, Private space of Self. Essential Bibliography: Milgram, S. (1971) *The Individual in a Social World.* Addison and Wesley, Reading.

Transformation In 'K' and Evolution in 'O' (W.R. Bion): See under *Evolution in 'O'* in the Glossary.

Transitional Object (D.W. Winnicott): Winnicott has said that between 4 and 18 months of age a single object (for example a bedcover) can take on a vital importance for a baby, especially at the moment of going to sleep, and he has called this object a 'transitional object'. It represents the baby's 'first non-me possession'. The transitional object is in the first place a real object, but at the same time it is a substitute maternal symbol. By the intense phantasy activity which it promotes and carries, the transitional object is situated in that intermediate area of experience which will have the task of maintaining external and internal reality separate and yet correlated all through life. In particular Winnicott says that what matters is not the object used but the use the baby makes of it; and that with growth the transitional object becomes de-cathected, but rather than being forgotten, it loses importance because its area is diffused into play, artistic creativity, religious feeling and dreams (see Ferretti 1990, pp.517–519). Associated Notions: Transitional phase, Group as object-Self, Group illusion, The group's common space. Essential Bibliography: Kaës, R. (1976) *L'appareil psychique groupal: Constructions du groupe.* Dunod, Paris.

Transitional Phase (D.W. Winnicott): Winnicott has defined as 'transitional' the phase of development in which the baby does not feel completely distinct from the object, but no longer feels it as part of its own body. The term 'transitional' refers, more precisely, to the idea of something lying between the subjective and the objective, which shows the gradual movement from the infant's illusion of itself creating the breast and the consequence of this delusion. (see Ferretti 1990). Associated Notions: Group illusion, Group-world, Transitional object, Presence of the group, Syncretic sociality. Essential Bibliography: Winnicott, D.W. (1965) *The Maturational Processes and the Facilitating Environment.* Hogarth Press, London. Reprinted, Karnac Books, London, 1995.

Transpersonal Diffusion: The term designates a particular form of transmission of mental states which pass from the individual to the group field. Mental states which are the object of transpersonal diffusion are not transmitted intentionally, but are diffused as a gas might be through the barriers formed by individuals' 'mental skin' and by group boundaries. Transpersonal diffusion is a particular form of commuting. Associated Notions: Commuting, Psychic transmission, Transpsychic transmission. Essential Bibliography: Winnicott, D.W. (1969) 'Mother's madness appearing in the clinical material as an Ego-alien factor.' In P.L. Giovacchini (ed.) *Tactics and Techniques in Psychoanalytic Psychotherapy.* Jason Aronson, Northvale, NJ.

Transpersonal Phenomena: In day-to-day language the expression 'interpersonal relations' is in current use to indicate relationships between people. The expression 'transpersonal phenomenon' indicates a different sort of phenomenon, which cannot be directly related either to persons or to interpersonal relations. However, these phenomena interfere both with people and with their relationships (see A. Bruni and G. Nebbiosi 1987). Associated Notions: Atmosphere, Medium, Primitive mentality. Essential Bibliography: Freud, S. (1926) *Address to the Society of B'nai B'rith.* SEXX.

Transpsychic Transmission: R. Kaës (1993, p.21) notes that what is transmitted between subjects, 'intersubjective transmission', is not of the same order as that which is transmitted through them, which is 'transpsychic transmission'. In fact, when there is communication between subjects, there is an obstacle, represented by the person with whom one is speaking, and there is also some experience of the separation between oneself and the other. In transpsychic transmission, on the other hand, these two obstacles disappear in favour of the demands of narcissism. More generally, Kaës emphasises the idea that 'transpsychic transmission' presupposes the abolition of subjective boundaries and space, while in 'intersubjective transmission' these elements are preserved. Associated Notions: Transpersonal diffusion, Transpersonal phenomena, Psychic transmission. Essential Bibliography: Bonaminio, V. *et al.* (1993) 'Le fantasie inconscie dei genitori come fattori ego-alieni nelle identificazioni del bambino.' *Rivista di Psicoanalisi 39*, 4; Kaës, R. *et al.* (1993) *Transmission de la vie psychique entre generations.* Dunod, Paris.

Valency (W.R. Bion): As Fornari (1981, p.186) points out: 'Bion rejects the libidinal theory of collectivity, replacing the concept of libido with that of valency, a term with no affective connotations.' A second characteristic of valency is its automatic nature. On this subject Bion (1961, p.185) writes: 'Although I use this term [valency] to express phenomena which appear as psychological facts or can be deduced from them, I should still like to use it to indicate availability at levels which are difficult to call mental; in fact they are characterised by the presence in man of behaviour more like the tropism of plants than motivated behaviour.' Associated Notions: Basic assumptions, Transpersonal diffusion. Essential Bibliography: Bion, W.R. (1961) *Experiences in Groups.* Karnac Books, London, 1968.

Waiting for the Messiah (W.R. Bion): Waiting for the Messiah means both the basic assumption of coupling, and the 'primitive stage' of group life. The term 'Messianic' indicates a characteristic of this type of waiting, which is charged with the hope of a future change, which will concern not only the individual person, but the entire group. In therapeutic groups, the hope for the Messiah is centred above all on phantasies of cure. Messianic hope, present in the small analytic group, may become an indefinite waiting, or else be placed on a fixed horizon; in this case it is an important factor of positive changes. Associated Notions: Group illusion, Emerging state of the group. Essential Bibliography: Bion, W.R. (1970) *Attention and Interpretation.* Karnac Books, London, 1988; Scholem, G. (1960) *On the Kabbalah and its Symbolism.* Schoken Books, New York.

Work-Group (W.R. Bion): The 'work-group', described by Bion in *Experiences in Groups,* represents a level and a function which are always present in the group. It is opposed to and coexistent with 'primitive mentality' and 'basic assumptions'. It refers to the purposes for which people join in groups, and therefore is based on the conscious and rational cooperation of the participants. It plays a part in the mental functioning of the group comparable to the 'Ego' of the individual psyche (see Fornari 1981, p.652). Associated Notions: Function-experience and function-institution, Organised group. Essential Bibliography: Bernabei, M. *et al.* (1987) 'Alcune osservazioni su gruppo di lavoro e assunti di base.' In C. Neri *et al.* (eds.) *Letture bioniane.* Borla, Rome.

Working Through: (Corresponding to German '*Durcharbeiten*'), in English 'working through' was described by Freud (1914) in these words: 'We must give the patient the time to immerse himself in that resistance which is now known to him, to work it through and overcome it.' In the psychoanalytical technique inspired by Melanie Klein, working through occupies a central position, and is entrusted not only to the patient, but also to the analyst. In group analysis working through is the result of co-operation between members, the analyst and the group as a collective subject. Associated Notions: α-Function , γ-Function. Essential Bibliography: Freud, S. (1914) *On Narcissism: An Introduction.* SE XIV.

World of ID (L.C. Knights): 'The things which really concern us are obviously those with which we are in personal and direct relations...these belong to the world which Martin Buber has defined as the world of Ego and Tu, the world of relationships. But man cannot live exclusively in the world of Tu; there is also the world of the neutral Id [it], the world which can be, and must be, manipulated and arranged, and which necessarily influences the quality of the personal world' (Knights 1971, p.30). Associated Notions: The group's common space. Essential Bibliography: Melchiori, G. (1973) *L'uomo e il potere*. Einaudi, Turin.

Bibliography

Aebischer, V. and Oberl, D. (1990) *Le Groupe en Psychologie Sociale.* Paris: Bordas-Dunod.

Agosta, F. (1988) 'Pensare in gruppo'. *Gruppo e Funzione Analitica, IX,* 3, 227–236.

Amabili, B. (1993) 'O: pensiero rappresentato da un segno, cornice di un punto espanso'. In M. Bernabei, Neri C. (eds.) Monographic number dedicated to the symbol: in Bion, Metaxù, 16, 49–53.

Amati, Sas S. (1977) 'Qualche riflessione sulla tortura per introdurre una discussione psicoanalitica'. *Rivista di Psicoanalisi, XXIII,* 3, 461–478.

Americo, A. (1983) 'Alcune osservazioni relative al costituirsi dell'area di appartenenza nell'ambito dei soggiorni estivi organizzati da un Centro Igiene Mentale'. *Gruppo e Funzione Analitica, IV,* 2–3, 91–97.

Ammaniti, M. and Fraire M. (1982) 'Il gruppo terapeutico nel trattamento istituzionale della psicosi'. *Gruppo e Funzione Analitica, III,* 3, 47–58.

Anzieu, D. (1976) *Le Groupe et l'Inconscient.* Paris: Bordas-Dunod.

Anzieu, D. (1981) *Le Groupe et l'Inconscient. L'imaginaire Groupal* (Second Edition). Paris: Dunod.

Anzieu, D. (1985) *Le moi-peau.* Paris: Bordas.

Anzieu, D. (1986) 'Cadre psychanalytique et enveloppes psychiques'. *Journal de la Psychanalyse de l'Enfant,* 12–24.

Anzieu, D. (1988) 'Introduction.' In D. Rosenfeld, *Psychoanalysis and Group.* London: Karnac Books.

Anzieu, D. and Martin, J.Y. (1968–86) *La Dynamique des Groupes Restreints.* Paris: PUF.

Arendt, H. (1963) *Eichmann in Jerusalem: A Report on the Banality of Evil.* New York:Viking Press.

Aulagnier, P. (1975) *La Violence de l'Interpretation. Du pictogramme à l'énancé.* Paris: PUF.

Badolato, C. and Di Iullo M.G. (1978) *Gruppi Terapeutici e Gruppi di Formazione.* Rome: Bulzoni.

Bakhtin, M.M. (1981) 'Forms of Time and Chronotope in the Novel' In *The Dialogic Imagination: Four Essays by M.M. Bakhtin.* Austin: University of Texas Press.

Bakhtin, M.M. (1984) *Problems of Dostoevsky's Poetics.* Manchester, MI: University of Manchester Press.

Baranger, M. and Baranger W. (1961–1962) 'La situacin analitica como campo dinmico'. *Revista Uruguaya de Psicoanlisis, 4,* 1, 3–54.

Baranger, M. and Baranger, W. (1969) *Problemas del campo psicanlitico.* Buenos Aires: Kargieman.

Barn, C.A. (1993) 'Esperienze di Supervisione nei Servizi'. *Quaderni di Koinos, 3,* 39–57, Rome: Borla, 1995.

Bateson, G. (1972) *Steps to an Ecology of Mind.* San Francisco: Chandler Publishing Company.

Bauleo, A.J. (ed.) (1974) *Los Sintomas de la Salud.* Buenos Aires: Cuarto Mondo.

Bauman, Z. (1989) *Modernity and the Holocaust.* Oxford: Basil Blackwell.

Bejarano, A. (1972) 'Resistance et transfert dans les groupes'. In D. Anzieu, A. Bejarano, R. Kaës, A. Missenard and J.B. Pontalis (eds.) *Le Travail Psychoanalytique dans les Groupes.* Paris: Dunod.

Benjamin, W. (1919) 'Die Aufgabe des bersetzers'. In *Gesammelte Schriften, IV,* 1, Frankfurt a. Main: Suhrkamp Verlag, 1972.

Benjamin, W. (1931) 'Kleine Geschichte der photographie'. In *Gesammelte Schriften I,* 2, Frankfurt a Main: Suhrkamp Verlag, 1974 .

Benjamin, W. (1933) 'Ber das mimetische Vermgen'. In *Gesammelte Schriften, II,* 1, Frankfurt a. Main: Suhrkamp Verlag, 1977.

Beradt, C. (1966) *Das Dritte Reich des Traums.* Munchen: Nympherburger Verlag.

Bernabei, M. *et al.* (1987) 'Alcune osservazioni su gruppo di lavoro e assunti di base'. In C. Neri *et al.* (eds.) *Letture Bioniane.* Rome: Borla.

Bernabei, M. (1994) 'Fattori terapeutici nei gruppi a termine: la funzione iniziatica. Fattori terapeutici nei gruppi e nelle istituzioni'. *Quaderni di Koinos, 2* (Edited by C. Neri, A., Correale and S. Contorni). Rome: Borla.

Bernabei, M. (1995) 'Il passaggio iniziatico: un fattore terapeutico nei gruppi a termine'. *Quaderni di Koinos, 2,* 195–208. Rome: Borla.

Bernabei, M. and Neri, C. (eds.) (1993) 'Monographic number dedicated to the symbol' in Bion. *Metaxù, XVI,* 7–13.

Bettelheim, B. (1966) 'Nachwort'. In C. Beradt, *Das Dritte Reich des Traums.* Munich: Nympherburger Verlag.

Bezoari, M. and Ferro, A. (1991) 'Percorsi nel campo bi-personale dell'analisi'. *Rivista di Psicoanalisi, XXXVII,* 1, 5–46.

Bick, E. (1968) *The Experience of the Skin in Early Object-Relations.* London: Karnac Books.

Bion ,W.R. (1962a) 'A theory of thinking'. *International Journal of Psycho-Analysis, 43,* 306–310.

Bion, W.R. (1962b) *Learning from Experience.* London: Karnac Books.

Bion, W.R. (1963) *Elements of Psychoanalysis.* London: Karnac Books.

Bion, W.R. (1967) *Second Thought (Selected Papers of Psychoanalysis).* London: Karnac Books.

Bion, W.R. (1970) *Attention and Interpretation.* London: Karnac Books.

Bion, W.R. (1977) 'Catastrophic change'. *Bulletin of British Psycho-Analytic Society, 5.*

Bion, W.R. (1987) *Clinical Seminars and Four Papers.* London: Karnac Books.

Bion, W.R. (1991) *A Memoir of the Future. Book One: The Dream.* London: Karnac Books.

Bion, W.R. (1992) *Cogitations.* London: Karnac Books.

Bion Talamo, P. (1991) 'Aggressivit, bellicosit, belligeranza'. Paper presented at the Centro Psicoanalitico di Torino. Unpublished.

Bleger, J. (1966a) 'Psychanalyse du cadre psychanalytique'. In R Kaës *et al.* (eds.) (1979) *Crise, Rupture et Dépassement. Introduction à L'analyse transitionelle.* Paris: Dunod.

Bleger, J. (1967a) 'Psychoanalysis of the psychoanalytic form.' *International Journal of Psycho-Analysis,* 1967a, 48, 511–519.

Bleger, J. (1966b) *Psico-higiene y Psicología. Institutional.* Buenos Aires: Paidós.

Bleger, J. (1967b) *Simbiosis y Ambigudad.* Buenos Aires: Paidós. English edition: *International Journal of Psychoanalysis,* 1967a, 48, pp.511–519.

Bleger, J. (1970) 'El grupo como institucion y el grupo en las instituciones'. In *Temas de Psicologia.* Buenos Aires: Nueva Visión.

Boas, F. (1911) *The Mind of Primitive Man.* New York: The McMillan Company.

Boccanegra, L. (1994) Intervento al Convegno – Incontro con René Kaës. I Fattori Terapeutici nei Gruppi. Rome, 21 May1994.

Bodei, R. (1991) *Geometria delle Passioni. Paura, Speranza, Felicit: Filosofia ed Uso Politico.* Milan: Feltrinelli.

Bonaminio, V., Di Renzo M.A. and Giannotti, A. (1993) 'Le fantasie inconsce dei genitori come fattori Ego alieni nelle identificazioni del bambino. Qualche riflessione su identit e falso Sé attraverso il materiale clinico dell'analisi infantile'. *Rivista di Psicoanalisi, XXXIX,* 4, 681–708.

Bonazza, M. (1993) 'Il gruppo di supervisione'. PhD Thesis in Psychology. Rome.

Bonfantini, M.A. and Grazia, R. (1976) 'Teoria della conoscenza e funzione dellicona in peirce'. *Versus: Quaderni di Studi Semiotici, 15,* 1.

Borges, J. L. (1970) *El Informe de Brodie.* In Obras Completas, E mecé Editores, Buenos Aires.

Borgogno, F. (1977) 'Teoria e tecnica del gruppo eterocentrato'. *Psicoterapia e Scienze Umane, 1,* 25–38.

Bowlby, J. (1969) 'Attachment'. In *Attachment and Loss,* Vol. I. New York: Basic Books.

Bowlby, J. (1988) *A Secure Base.* London: Routledge.

Bria, P. (1986) 'Individuo, gruppo e matrice di base della socialità. Una riflessione sul gruppo in termini di bi-logica'. *Archivio di Psicologia, Neurologia, Psichiatria, XLVI,* 3–4.

Brown, D., Pedder, J. (1979) *Introduction to Psychotherapy* (Second Edition) London: Tavistock-Routledge, 1991.

Bruni, A. (1985) 'Il gruppo che non c'e: un riferimento sulla separazione (nota 1a)'. *Gruppo e Funzione Analitica, VI*, 1, 41–47.

Bruni, A. and Nebbiosi G. (1987) 'Colloquio con K. Pribram'. *Gruppo e Funzione Analitica, VIII*, 1, 79–90.

Brutti, C. and Parlani, R. (1983) 'Sulla bugia. Appunti per una ricerca psicoanalitica'. *Gruppo e Funzione Analitica, IV*, 1, 51–53.

Calvino, I. (1964) 'Tutto in un punto'. In *Le Cosmicomiche*, Torino: Einaudi, 1965.

Camaioni, L. (1980) 'La prima infanzia'. Bologna: Il Mulino.

Canetti, E. (1960) *Masse und Macht*. Hamburg: Claassen Verlag.

Carli, R. (1993) *Introduction to D. Rosenfeld, Psicoanalisi e Gruppi – Storia e Dialettica*. Roma: Borla.

Cavafy, C.P. (1992) 'Waiting for the barbarians.' In *Collected Poems*. Cambridge, MA: Princeton University Press.

Chomsky, N. (1977) *Dialogues avec Mitsou Ronat*. Paris: Flammarion.

Cinciripini, C. and Di Leone, G. (1990) 'Circolazione degli affetti nel gruppo dei curanti di una cooperativa per l'assistenza'. *Gruppo e Funzione Analitica, XI*, 3, 33–38.

Cinti, D. (1989) *Dizionario Mitologico*. Milan: Sonzogno.

Corrao, F. (1977) 'Per una topologia analitica'. *Rivista di Psicoanalisi, XXIII*, 1, 20–43.

Corrao, F. (1981) 'Struttura poliadica e funzione gamma'. *Gruppo e Funzione Analitica, II*, 2, 25–31

Corrao, F. (1982) 'Psicoanalisi e ricerca di gruppo'. *Gruppo e Funzione Analitica, III*, 3, 23–27.

Corrao, F. (1985) 'Il senso dell'analisi (Teoria e prassi dell'evento. Nota II)'. *Gruppo e Funzione Analitica, VI*, 2, 9–18.

Corrao, F. (1986) 'Il concetto di campo come modello teorico'. *Gruppo e Funzione Analitica, VII*, 1, 9–21.

Corrao, F. (1992) Modelli psicoanalitici: mito, passione, memoria. Roma-Bari: Laterza.

Corrao, F. (1994) 'Duale <=> Gruppale'. In G. Di Chiara and C. Neri (eds.) *Psicoanalisi Futura*. Rome: Borla.

Corrao, F. and Neri, C. (1981) 'Introduction'. Monographic Number of the Italian Psychoanalytical Review Dedicated to the Work of W. R. Bion, (Edited by Partenope Bion Talamo and Claudio Neri), XXVII, 3–4, 363–367.

Correale, A. and Parisi, M. (1979) Aspetti della depersonalizzazione nel gruppo. *Gruppo e Funzione Analitica, I*, 1, 57–60.

Correale, A. (1986) 'Depersonalizzazione e percezione spaziale in gruppo'. *Gruppo e Funzione Analitica, VII*, 1, 81–89.

Correale, A. (1987) 'Ps <=> D'. In C. Neri *et al.* (ed.) *Letture Bioniane*. Rome: Borla.

Correale, A. (1991) *Il Campo Istituzionale*. Rome: Borla.

Correale, A. (1992) *Campo (Modello di) Interazioni*, n.0, 124–126.

Corrente, G. (1992) 'Trasformazioni del campo <=> identité. *Koinos, XIII*, 2, 67–72.

Cotinaud, O. (1976) *Groupe et Analyse Institutionelle*. Paris: Ed. du Centurion.

Cruciani, P. (1983) 'Sighele, Le Bon, Trotter e McDougall: le fonti di Psicologia delle masse'. In C. Neri (ed.) *Prospettive della Ricerca Psicoanalitica di Gruppo*. Rome: Kappa.

Cuomo, G. (1986) 'La prospettiva gruppale in psicoterapia: il paziente silenzioso'. In *AA.VV., Modelli Psicologici e Psicoterapia*. Rome: Bulzoni.

Cupelloni, P. (1983) Contributo al dibattito del convegno sulle microallucinazioni. *Gruppo e Funzione Analitica, IV*, 1, 75–82.

D'Apruzzo, A. (1987) 'Funzione alfa ed elementi beta'. In C. Neri *et al.* (eds.) *Letture Bioniane*. Rome: Borla.

Dazzi, N. (1987) 'Note sulla lettura dell'opera di Bion W.R.' In C. Neri *et al.* (eds.) *Letture Bioniane*. Rome: Borla.

De Lillo, D. (1991) *MAO II*. New York: Vintage.

De Martis, D. and Barale, F. (1993) 'Dinamiche di gruppo e istituzione universitaria'. In R. Contardi, R. Gaburri, S. Vender (eds.) *I Fattori Terapeutici nei Gruppi e nelle Istituzioni.* Rome: Borla.

De Risio, S. (1986) 'Dinamiche individuo-gruppo'. *Rivista Italiana di Gruppo-Analisi, II.*

De Simone, G. (1981) 'Note sul setting di gruppo'. *Gruppo e Funzione Analitica, II,* 3, 13–17.

Dell'Anna, G. (1993) 'La membrana: una metafora delle organizzazioni psichiche di confinamento'. Degree Thesis in Psychology, Rome.

Di Chiara, G. (1992) 'Tre fattori fondamentali della esperienza psicoanalitica: lincontro, il racconto e il commiato'. In A. Robutti and L. Nissim (eds.) *Antologia.* Milan: Cortina.

Di Leone, G. (1991) Intervento al Convegno su: Gruppo di ricerca sull'uso del piccolo gruppo nelle istituzioni psichiatriche della UOT 7, USL RM 3.

Di Leone, G. (1993) 'Illusione e Affetti'. Presentation at Convegno: I Fattori Terapeutici nel Gruppo e nelle Istituzioni, Roma.

Di Norscia, G., Tessari G. (1986) 'Vicissitudini di un gruppo di operatori in ambito istituzionale'. *Gruppo e Funzione Analitica, VII,* 2, 137–141.

Di Trapani, R., Gentile, C.M., Marchetta, E. and Moggi, D. (1994) 'Il gruppo e la memoria: ostruzioni e costruzioni'. Prize presentation of Francesco Corrao, Palermo.

Dicks, H.V. (1977) *Marital Tensions.* New York: Basic Books.

Dostoevsky, F. (1880) *Karamazov Bratja.* [The Brothers Karamazov]

Durkheim, E. (1893) *Les Regles de la Methode Sociologique.* Paris: Alcan (new edition, 1947, Paris: PUF).

Durkheim, E. (1897) *Le Suicide. Etude de Sociologie.* Paris: Alcan.

Durkheim, E. (1901) *Sociologie et Sciences Sociales. De la Methode dans les Sciences.* Paris: Alcan.

Einstein, A. and Infeld, L. (1938) ['Die evolution der physik'. Werner Preusser, Wien Zsolnay, 1950. The evolution of Physics. The growth of ideas from early concepts to relativity and quanta.]

Ezriel, H. (1950) 'A psychoanalytic approach to group treatment'. *British Journal of Medical Psychology, 23,* 59–74.

Ezriel, H. (1952) 'Notes on psycho-analytic group therapy: II. Interpretations and research'. *Psychiatry, 15.*

Ezriel, H. (1973) 'Psychoanalytic group therapy'. In L.R. Wolberg and E.K. Schwartz, *Group Therapy: An Overview.* New York: International Medical Books.

Fachinelli, E. (1983) *Claustrofilia: Saggio sull'Orologio Telepatico in Psicoanalisi.* Milan: Feltrinelli.

Fadda, P. (1984) 'Il ruolo della teoria del pensiero nel passaggio dal gruppo di lavoro specializzato al rapporto tra mistico e istituzione'. PhD Thesis in Psychology, Rome.

Falci, A. (1990) 'Tra costrizione e rivelazione: le passioni come forme creative'. *Gruppo e Funzione Analitica, XI,* 2, 74–83.

Ferretti, E. (1990) 'Sogno, s, area transizionale: lineamenti speculativi sull'analista al lavoro per prospettive di ricerca'. *Rivista di Psicoanalisi, XXXVI,* 3, 517–559.

Ferruta, A. (1992) Intervento al Convegno su: Genius loci: una funzione del gruppo analoga a quella della divinit tutelare di un luogo, Milan.

Figà Talamanca, A. (1991) 'Modelli semplici di spazio'. *Koinos, XII,* 2, 115–133.

Fischer, G.N. (1987) *Les Concepts Fondamentaux de la Psychologie Sociale.* Paris: Bordas.

Fornari, F. (1971) 'Pour une psychanalyse des institutions'. In R. Kaës *et al.* (1980), *L'Institution et les Institutions.* Paris: Dunod, .

Fornari, F. (1981) *From Freud to Bion.* Monographic Number of the Italian Psychoanalytical Review Dedicated to the Work of W. R. Bion, (Edited by Parthenope Bion Talamo and Claudio Neri), XXVII, 3–4, 662–672.

Fornari, F. (1987) 'Gruppo e codici oggettivi.' In G. Trentini (ed.) *Il Cerchio Magico.* Milan: F. Angeli.

Foulkes, S.H. (1948) *Introduction to Group-Analytic Psychotherapy: Studies in the Social Integration of Individuals and Groups.* London: Heinemann.

Foulkes, S.H. (1964) *Therapeutic Group Analysis.* London: George Allen & Unwin.

Foulkes, S.H. (1975) *Group-Analytic Psychotherapy: Methods and Principles.* London: Gordon & Breach.

Foulkes, S.H. and Anthony, E.J. (1957) *Group Psychotherapy: The Psychoanalitical Approach.* London: Penguin Books, [1965].

Freud, S. (1899) *ber Deckerinnerungen.* Gesammelte Werke, 1, Fischer Verlag, Frankfurt am Main, 1940–1950. [*Screen Memories.* Standard Edition, vol. 3, The Hogarth Press (1953–74), London].

Freud, S. (1900) *Die Traumdeutung.* Gesammelte Werke, 2/3, Fischer Verlag, Frankfurt am Main, 1940–1950. [*The Interpretation of Dreams.* Standard Edition vol. 4, The Hogarth Press (1953–74), London].

Freud, S. (1912–13) *Totem und Tabu.* Gesammelte Werke, 9, Fischer Verlag, Frankfurt am Main, 1940–1950.[*Totem and Taboo.* Standard Edition, vol. 13, The Hogarth Press (1953–74), London].

Freud, S. (1914) *Zur Einfhrung des Narzissmus.* Gesammelte Werke, 10, Fischer Verlag, Frankfurt am Main, 1940–1950. [*On Narcissism. An introduction.* Standard Edition, vol. 14, The Hogarth Press (1953–74), London].

Freud, S. (1921) *Massenpsychologie und Ich-Analyse.* Gesammelte Werke, 13, Fischer Verlag, Frankfurt am Main, 1940–1950. [*Group Psychology and the Analysis of Ego.* Standard Edition, vol. 18, The Hogarth Press (1953–74), London].

Freud, S. (1926–1941) *Ansprache an die Mitglieder des vereins Bnai Brith.* Gesammelte Werke, 17, Fischer Verlag, Frankfurt am Main, 1940–1950. [*Address to the Society of Bnai Brith.* Standard Edition, vol. 20, The Hogarth Press (1953–74), London].

Gaburri, E. (1986) 'Disturbi del pensiero e identit tra l'individuo e il gruppo'. *Gruppo e Funzione Analitica, VII*, 2, 111–121.

Gaburri, E. (1992) 'Emozioni, Affetti, Personificazioni'. *Rivista di Psicoanalisi, XXXVIII*, 2, 325–351.

Gaburri, E. and Contardi, R.D. (1993) 'Evoluzione storica e paradigma attuale dei fattori inibitori/ evolutivi nel gruppo'. In R. Contardi, G. Gaburri, S. Vender, *Fattori Terapeutici nei Gruppi e nelle Istituzioni.* Rome: Borla.

Galanter, M. (1989) *Cults Faith, Healing and Coercion.* Oxford: Oxford University Press.

Gear, M.C. and Liendo, E.C. (1979) *Psicoterapia de la Pareja y Grupo Familiar con Orientacin Psicoanlitica.* Buenos Aires: Galerna.

Giannakoulas, A. (1992) 'La membrana diadica'. *Interazioni, n. 0*, 129–132.

Gluckman, M. (1965) *Politics, Law and Ritual in Tribal Society.* New York: The New American Library, 1968.

Gombrich, E.H. (1960) 'Freuds aesthetics'. *Encounter*, 30–40, 1966.

Goodall, J. (1990) *Through a Window. Thirty Years with the Chimpanzees of Gombe.* London: Soko Publications.

Granet, M. (1922) 'Le dépôt de l'enfant sur le sol. Rites anciens et ordalies mythiques'. In *Études Sociologiques sur la Chine,* Paris: PUF, 1953.

Grass, G. (1990) *The Tin Drum.* Bournemouth: Vintage Books.

Grinberg, L., Sor, D. and Tabak De Bianchedi, E. (1972) *Introducon a las Ideas de Bion. Grupos, Conocimiento, Psicosis, Pensamiento, Trasformaciones, Pratica Psicoanlitica.* Buenos Aires: Ediciones Nueva Visión.

Hall, E.T. (1966) *The Hidden Dimension.* New York: Doubleday.

Hautmann, G. (1985) 'Seminario analitico di gruppo come strumento di formazione'. *Gruppo e Funzione Analitica, VI*, 2, 49–56.

Hinshelwood, R. D. (1987) *What Happens in Groups.* London: Free Association Books.

Hobson, J.A., Spagna, T. and Earls, P. (1977) *Dreamstage. An Experimental Portrait of the Sleeping Brain.* USA: Hoffmann-La Roche Inc.

Holmes, J. (1993) *John Bowlby and Attachment Theory.* London: Routledge.

Hubermann, L.E. (1994) (Personal communication).

Imbasciati, A. (1991) *Affetto e Rappresentazione: per una Psicoanalisi dei Processi Cognitivi.* Milan: F. Angeli.

Jaffé R. (1992) 'Relazioni emotive dal gruppo terapeutico al gruppo di supervisione: un'esperienza in un'istituzione'. *Koinos, XIII*, 1, 105–115.

Jannuzzi, G. (1979) 'Scena primaria, contratto e scena escatologica nel "qui ed ora" del gruppo analitico'. *Gruppo e Funzione Analitica, I,* 1, 61–70.

Jaques, E. (1955) 'Social systems as defense against persecutory and depressive anxiety'. In M. Klein, P. Heimann, R. Money-Kyrle (eds.) *New Directions in Psychoanalysis.* London: Tavistock Publications.

Jung, C.G. (1912) 'Symbole der wandlung. Analyse des vorspiels zu einer schizophrenie'. In Gesammelte Werke, 5, Rascher Verlag, Zurich-Stuttgart. Symbols of Trasformation. *An Analysis of the Prelude to a Case of Schizophrenia. The Collected Works of C.G. Jung, Vol 5,* Routledge & Kegan Paul, London.

Jung, C.G. (1928) *Die Beziehungen Zwischen dem Ich und dem Unbewussten.* Gesammelte Werke, 7, Rascher Verlag, Zurich-Stuttgart. [*The Relations Between the Ego and the Unconscious.* The Collected Works of Jung C.G., vol. 7, Routledge & Kegan Paul, London].

Jung, C.G. (1948) *Vorwort Zum I Ging.* Gesammelte Werke, 11, Rascher Verlag, Zurich-Stuttgart. [*Foreword to the I Ching.* The Collected Works of Jung C.G., vol. 11, Routledge & Kegan Paul, London].

Kaës, R. (1976) *L'Appareil Psychique Groupal. Constructions du Groupe.* Paris: Dunod.

Kaës, R. (1985) 'Le groupe comme appareil de transformation'. *Revue de Psychothérapie et Psychanalyse de Groupe,* 5–6, 91–100.

Kaës, R. (1993) *Le Groupe et le Sujet du Groupe.* Paris: Dunod.

Kaës, R. (1994) *La Parole et le Lien. Processus Associatifs dans les Groupes.* Paris: Dunod.

Kaës, R., Faimberg, H. *et al.* (1993) *Transmission de la vie Psychique entre Gnrations.* Paris: Dunod.

Khan, M.M.R. (1974) *The Privacy of Self.* New York: International Universities Press.

Knights, L.C. (1971) *Public Voices: Literature and Politics with Special Reference to the Seventeenth Century.* Totowa, NJ: Rowman and Littlefield.

Kohut, H. (1971) *The Analysis of the Self.* London: Hogarth Press.

Kohut, H. (1978) *The Search for the Self. Selected Writings of Heinz Kohut 1950–1978.* (Ed.) Paul H. Ornstein) New York: International University Press.

Kohut, H. (1984) *How Does Analysis Cure?* Chicago: Chicago University Press.

Koiré, A. (1948) 'Du mond de l «a-peu-près» l'univers de la précision'. In *Études d'Histoire de la Pensée Philosophique.* Paris: Armand Colin.

Kuhn, T.S. (1962) *The Structure of Scientific Revolutions.* Chicago: University of Chicago Press.

La Forgia, M. (1992) 'La sincronicità. In A. Carotenuto *Trattato di Psicologia Analitica.* Torino: UTET.

Lacan, J. (1949) 'Le stade du miroir comme formateur de la fonction du Je'. In *Ecrits. Vol. I.* Paris: Edition du Seuil.

Lakoff, G. and Johnson, M. (1980) *Metaphors We Live By.* Chicago: Chicago University Press.

Laplanche, J., Pontalis J.B. (1967) *Vocabulaire de la Psychanalyse.* Paris: PUF.

Larousse, P. (1896) *Nouveau Dictonnaire Illustré.* Paris: Larousse

Le Bon, G. (1895) *Psichologie des Foules.* Paris: PUF,1990.

Lévy Bruhl L. (1922) *La Mentalité Primitive.* Paris: PUF.

Lewin, K. (1936) *Principles of Topological Psychology.* New York: McGraw-Hill.

Lewin, K. (1948) *Resolving Social Conflicts.* New York: Harper.

Lewin, K. (1951) *Field Theory in Social Science.* New York: Harper & Row.

Lichtenberg, J.D. (1983) *Psychoanalysis and Infant Research.* Hillsdale, NJ: The Analytic Press.

Lichtenberg, J.D. *et al.* (1992) *Self and Motivational System.* Hillsdale, NJ: The Analytic Press.

Lindauer, M. (1990) *Botschaft ohne Worte.* Munich: Piper GmbH.

Lo Verso, G. and Vinci, S. (1990) *Il Gruppo nel Lavoro Clinico: Bibliografia Ragionata.* Milan: Giuffrè.

Lo Verso, G. and Papa, M. (1992) 'Il gruppo come oggetto di conoscenza e la conoscenza del gruppo'. In F. Di Maria, G. Lo Verso (eds.) (1996) *Il Nodo e il Tondo. Teorie e Tecniche della Dinamica di Gruppo.* Roma: Cortina.

Longo, M. (1983) 'Foulkes e la gruppoanalisi'. In C. Neri (ed.) *Prospettive della Ricerca Psicoanalitica nel Gruppo.* Rome: Kappa.

Lotman, J.M. (1978) *Tekst v Tekste.* Tartu: Tartuskiij gos universitet, 1981.

Lotman, J.M. (1985) *La Semiosfera. L'Asimmetria e il Dialogo delle Strutture Pensanti.* Venice: Marsilio.

Lotman, J.M. (1990) *Universe of the Mind: A Semiotic Theory of Culture (Second World Series).* Bloomington, IN: Indiana University Press.

Lotman, J.M. (1993) *Kul'tura i Vryv.* Moscow: Gnosis.

Lucas, P. (1985) 'L'espace analityque des groupes thrapeutiques'. *Revue de Psychothrapie Psychoanalytique de Groupe,* 1–2, 119–133.

Lugones, M. (1994) 'Gioco e rappresentazione: Spiele, Lutspiel, Trauerspiel.' In AA.VV., Il transfert nella analisi dei bambini. Rome: Borla.

Luhmann, N. (1980) *Gesellschaftsstruktur und Semantik.* Frankfurt a. Main: Suhrkamp Verlag.

Mancia, M. (1996) *Sonno e sogno.* Rome-Bari: Laterza.

Mandel, G. (ed.) (1992) *Saggezza Islamica: le Novelle dei Sufi.* Milan: Edizioni Paoline.

Manfredi Turillazzi, S. (1974) 'Dalle interpretazioni mutative di Strachey alle interpretazioni delle relazioni degli oggetti interni'. *Rivista di Psicoanalisi, XX,* 9, 127–143.

Marais, E. N. (1921) *The Soul of the White Ant.* London: Methuen & Co.

Margherita, G. (1987) Supervisione in un servizio psichiatrico pubblico. *Gruppo e Funzione Analitica, VIII,* 3, 309–317.

Marinelli, S. (1991) 'Notazioni su diversi modi di concepire lo spazio mentale'. *Koinos, XII,* 2, 69–77.

Marinelli, S. (1993) *Presentato al Convegno su: Brain: Pensiero di Gruppo.* Rome: Centro Ricerche Psicoanalitiche di Gruppo.

Marramao, G. (1992) *Kairs. Apologia del Tempo Debito.* Rome-Bari: Laterza.

Massa, R. (1979) 'Il ruolo degli ormoni steroidei nel controllo del comportamento socio sessuale dei vertebrati'. In V. Parisi, F. Robustelli (eds.)(1982) *Il Dibattito sulla Sociobiologia: Atti del 1 Seminario sulla Sociobiologia.* Rome: CNR.

McDougall, M. (1927) *The Group Mind.* London: Cambridge University Press.

McLean, P.D. (1970) 'The triune brain, emotion and scientific bias.' In F. Schmidt (ed.) The *Neurosciences, Second Study Program.* Rockefeller University Press.

McLuhan, M. (1977) *From the Eye to the Ear.* New York: Harcourt Brace.

Melchiorri, G. (1973) *L'Uomo e il Potere.* Torino: Einaudi.

Meltzer, D. (1984) *La Vita Onirica. Una Revisione della Teoria della Tecnica Psicoanalitica.* Rome: Borla, 1989.

Meltzer, D. (1992) *The Claustrum. An Investigation of Claustrophobic Phenomena.* Cambridge: The Roland Harris Education Trust.

Menarini, R. and Pontalti, C. 'Il modello foulkesiano di matrice e terapia analitica di gruppo'. In G. Lo Verso and G. Venza (eds.) *Cultura e Tecniche di Gruppo nel Lavoro Clinico e Sociale in Psicologia.* Rome: Bulzoni, 1984.

Meotti, F. (1980) 'Contributo alla riflessione psicoanalitica sul tempo'. *Rivista di Psicoanalisi, XXVI,* 1, 43–52.

Meotti, F. (1986) 'Elaborare'. *Rivista Italiana di Psicoanalisi, XXXII,* 2, 271–278.

Meslin, M. (1986) 'L'Hermneutique des rituel dinitiotion'. In J. Ries (ed.), *Les Rites d'Initiation.* Louvain-La Neuve: Centre d'Histoire des Religions.

Metter, I. (1992) [1994] *Geneologia.* Turin: Einowdi.

Milgram, S. (1971) *The Individual in a Social World.* Reading: Addison and Wesley.

Missenard, A. (1989) Un eloquent silence: remarques sur le transfert/contretransfert. Intervention au congrs dAuxerre.

Mobasser, E. (1992) 'Identità funzionale nel gruppo'. *Koinos, XIII,* 2, 53–60.

Montaigne, M.E. (1957) *The Complete Works of Montaigne. Essays, Travel Journal, Letters.* Stanford: Stanford University Press.

Moreno, J. (1948) *Psychodrama.* New York: Beacon.

Moreno, J. (1954) *Who Shall Survive? Foundations of Sociometry, Group Psychotherapy and Sociodrama*. New York: Beacon House.

Murphy, G. (1951) *An Introduction to Psychology*. New York: Harper.

Napolitani, D. (1987) *Individualità e Gruppalità*. Torino: Boringhieri.

Narayan, R. K. (1973) *The Mahabharata : 1. The Book of the Beginning* (English translation J.A.B. van Buitenen, ed.) Chicago: The University of Chicago Press.

Neri, C. (1979a) 'La culla di spago'. *Quadrangolo, IV*, 1, 27–32.

Neri, C. (1979b) 'La torre di Babele: lingua, appartenenza, spazio-tempo nello stato gruppale nascente'. *Gruppo e Funzione Analitica, I*, 2–3, 25–47.

Neri, C. (1993) 'Campo: tre possibili impieghi e linee di sviluppo dell'idea in ambito psicoanalitico e psichiatrico'. *Psiche, I*, 2, 289–295.

Neri, C. (1993) 'Genius Loci: una funzione del luogo analoga a quella di una divinit tutelare'. *Koinos, XIV*, 1–2, 161–174.

Neri, C. (1994) 'Nomos: il diritto della Comunit dei fratelli'. In G. Di Chiara and C. Neri (eds.), *Psicoanalisi Futura*. Rome: Borla.

Neri, C. *et al.* (1990) *Fusionalità: Scritti di Psicoanalisi Clinica*. Rome: Borla.

Nicolosi, S. (1987) 'La configurazione contenitore-contenuto'. In C. Neri *et al.* (ed.), *Letture Bioniane*. Rome: Borla.

Pallier, L. (1992) 'Alcune considerazioni sulla mania in relazione ad una insufficiente strutturazione del Sé.' Presentato al Panel: *Sviluppi della ricerca sulla fusionalità*. Centro di Psicoanalisi Romano, Rome.

Palmieri, M.A. (1988) 'Il gruppo tra sentimento di non esistenza e di esistenza'. *Gruppo e Funzione Analitica, IX*, 3, 253–269.

Pasolini, P.P. (1956) 'Il pianto della scavatrice'. In *Le Ceneri di Gramsci*. Milan: Garzanti, 1957.

Pauletta, G. (ds) (1989) *Modelli Psicoanalitici nel Gruppo*. Milan: Cortina.

Peirce, C.S. (1878) 'Deduction, Induction and Hypothesis.' In (1931–35) *Collected Papers*. Cambridge: The Belknap Press of Harvard University.

Perelman, C., and Olbrechts Tyteca, L. (1958) *Traité de l'Argumentation. La Nouvelle Rhetorique*. Paris: PUF.

Perri, D. (1993) Intervention in the inaugural lecture at the *IIPG*. (Rome)

Perrotti, P. (1983) 'Eclissi dell'Io nel gruppo terapeutico'. In *La Processualit nel Gruppo*. Rome: Bulzoni.

Petrella, F. (1993) *Turbamenti Affettivi e Alterazioni dell'Esperienza*. Milan: Cortina.

Petrini, R. (1986) 'L'interpretazione come strutturazione e ristrutturazione nel campo mentale dell'analista'. *Gruppo e Funzione Analitica, VII*, 1, 90–94.

Petrolini, E. (1917) *Nerone*. In G. Antonucci (ed.) (1993) *Il Teatro di Petrolini*. Rome: Newton Compton.

Piaget, J. (1926) La Répresentation du Monde chez l'Enfant. Paris: Alcan.

Pichon-Rivière, E. (1977) *El Proceso Grupal. Del Psicoanlisè a la Psicologisa Social*. Buenos Aires: Nueva Visiòn.

Pines, M. (1984) 'Reflections on mirroring'. *International Review of Psycho-Analysis, II*, 27–42. Reprinted in M.Pines (1998) *Circular Reflections*. London: Jessica Kingsley Publishers.

Pomar, R. (1987) 'La congiunzione costante in Bion, W.R.' In C. Neri *et al.* (ed.) *Letture Bioniane*. Rome: Borla.

Pomar, R. (1994) Personal comunication.

Pribram, K.H. (1991) *Brain and Perception: Holonomy and Structure in Figural Processing*. Hillside: LFA.

Privat, P. and Chapelier, J.B. (1987) 'De la constitution d'un espace therapeutique groupal propos de groupes d'enfants à la latence'. *Revue de Psychotherapie Psychoanalytique de Group*, 7–8, 7–28.

Privat, J. and Privat, P. (1987) 'D'une utilisation particulière du jeu en groupe'. *Revue de Psychoterapie Psychanalytique de Groupe*, 7–8, 89–98.

Puget, J. *et al.* (1982) *El Grupo y sus Configuraciones*. Buenos Aires: Lugar ed.

Redl, F. (1942) 'Group, emotion and leadership'. *Psychiatry, V*, 573–6.

Reich, W. (1933) *Characteranalysise*. Copenhagen: Verlag für Sexualpolitik.

Resnik, S. (1983) 'L'individuo e il gruppo. Prima edizione di una lettura tenuta a Roma il 3/5/1982'. *Quaderni di Psicoterapia di Gruppo, 1* (1983) 11–23.

Riccio, D. (1987) 'Presentazione a "Letture Bioniane"'. *Gruppo e Funzione Analitica, VIII,* 2, 207–214.

Ries, J. (ed.) (1986) *Les Rites d'Initiation.* Louvain-la Neuve: Centre d'histoire des religions.

Rogers, C. (1970) *Carl Rogers on Encounter Groups.* New York: Harper.

Romano, R. (1986) 'Eventi, funzioni, transformazioni del campo di gruppo'. *Gruppo e Functione Analitica,* VII, 1, 30–41.

Rosenfeld, D. (1988) *Psychoanalysis and Groups.* London: Karnac Books.

Rouchy, J.C. (1980) 'Processus archaques et transfert en groupe-analyse'. *Connexions, 31,* 36–60.

Ruberti, L. (1990) 'La circolazione degli affetti nello spazio di un gruppo infantile'. *Gruppo e Funzione Analitica, X,* 1, 21–28.

Russo, L. (1993) 'L'importanza di Massenpsychologie nella definizione freudiana di "apparato psichico"'. *Koinos, XIV,* 1–2, 63–86.

Santi, P. (ed) (1989) *Repertorio di Musica Sinfonica.* Milan: Ricordi-Giunti.

Sarno, L. (1982) 'Memoria, linguaggio e conoscenza in Bion W.R. (prima parte)' *Gruppo e Funzione Analitica, III,* 2, 29–38.

Sarno, L. (1983) 'Memoria, linguaggio e conoscenza in Bion W.R. (seconda parte)' *Gruppo e Funzione Analitica, IV,* 2–3, 39–49.

Sartre, J.P. (1984; 1991) *Critique of Dialectical Reason,* vol.I; vol.II. London: Verso editions.

Scheidlinger, S. (1964) 'Identification, the sense of belonging and of identity in small group'. *International Journal of Group Psychotherapy, 14.*

Schilder, P. (1939) 'Results and problems of group psychotherapy in severe neurosis'. *Mental Hygene, 23.*

Schmitt, C. (1974) *Der Nomos der Erde im Völkerrecht des 'Jus Publicum Europaeum'.* Berlin: Dunker & Humblot.

Scholem, G. (1960) *Zur Kabbala und ihrer Simbolik.Wissenschaftliche Buchgesellschaft, Darmstadt.* On the kabbalah and its symbolism. New York: Schoken Books.

Searles, H.F. (1960) *The Nonhuman Environment.* Madison C.T. and New York: International University Press.

Searles, H.F. (1965) *Collected Papers on Schizofrenia and Related Subjects.* Madison C.T. and New York: International University Press.

Siani, P. (1992) *Psicologia del Sé: da Kohut alle Nuove Applicazioni Cliniche.* Torino: Bollati-Boringhieri.

Siracusano, F. (1986) 'L'esistenza ectopica del gruppo'. *Gruppo e Funzione Analitica, VII,* 1, 51–63.

Slavson, S.R. (1964) *A Textbook in Analytic Group Psychotherapy.* New York: International University Press.

Soavi, G.C. (1989) 'Sono pensieri le emozioni?' *Gruppo e Funzione Analitica, X,* 1, 7–20.

Solano, L. and Coda, R. (1994) *Relazioni, Emozioni, Salute. Introduzione a Psicoimmunologia.* Padua: Piccin.

Sommaruga, P. (1981) 'Il transfert nei piccoli gruppi.' *Gruppo e Funzione Analitica, II,* 3, 19–22.

Stern, D.N. (1985) *The Interpersonal World of the Infant.* New York: Basic Books.

Tagliacozzo, R. (1976) 'La depersonalizzazione crisi di rappresentazione del Sé nella realtà esterna'. *Rivista di Psicoanalisi, XXII,* 3, 322–332.

Tinbergen, N. (1953) *Social Behaviour in Animals.* London: Methuen & Co.

Trentini, G. (1987) 'Il gruppo come luogo della sorgente di omologazione intersoggettiva dei ruoli'. In *Il Cerchio Magico.* Milan: F. Angeli, 1987.

Turquet, P. (1975) 'Threats to identity in the large groups'. In L. Kreeger (ed.) *The Large Group: Dynamics and Therapy.* London: Constable.

Van Gennep, A. (1891) *Les Rites de Passage.* Paris: Nourry, 1909.

Vanni, F. (1984) *Modelli Mentali di Gruppo.* Milan: Cortina.

Vender, S. (1992) 'Esperienze nei gruppi di formazione alla relazione'. *Koinos, XII,* 1, 117–128.

Viderman, S. (1970) *La Construction de l'Espace Analytique.* Paris: Gallimard, 1982.

Vincent, J.D. (1986) *Biologie des Passions.* Paris: Editions Odile Jacob.

Viola, M. (1981) 'Fantasma originario, fantasia e rappresentazione in un gruppo analiticamente orientato'. *Gruppo e Funzione Analitica, II,* 3, 47–56.

Weber, M. (1988) *The Protestant Ethic and the Spirit of Capitalism* (2nd edition). Los Angeles: Roxburry Publishing Company.

Weil, S. (1941) *Oeuvres Complète, Vol. I.* Paris: Gallimard, 1991.

Whitaker, D.S. and Liebermann, M.A. (1964) *Psychotherapy Through Group Process.* New York: Atherton.

Whorf, B. L. (1956) *Language, Thought and Reality.* Cambridge, MA: MIT Press.

Winnicott, D.W. (1965) *Maturational Processes and the Facilitating Environment.* Madison C.T.., New York: International Universities Press.

Winnicott, D.W. (1969) *Mother's Madness Appearing in the Clinical Material as an Ego-alien Factor.* In C. Winnicott, R. Shepherd, M. Davis (ed.) (1989) *Psycho-Analytic Explorations.* London: Karnac Books.

Wittgenstein, L. (1919) 'Gespräche Über Freud.' In *Vorlesungen und Gespräche über Ästhetik, Psychologie und Religion,* VR Kleine, Vandenhoeck-Reihe, 1968. [Lectures and Conversations on Aesthetics, Psychology and Religious Belief. Ed. Cyril Barrett. Oxford: Blackwell, 1966].

Wolf, A. and Schwartz, E.K. (1962) *Psychoanalysis in Groups.* New York: Grune and Stratton.

Wolf, A. and Schwartz, E.K. (1970) *'See Beyond the Couch...'* New York: Science House.

Wolf, A. and Schwartz, E.K. (1972) 'Psychoanalysis in group'. In H.I. Kaplan and B.J. Sadok, *The Origins of Group Psychoanalysis.* New York: Aronson J.

Wolf, E.W. (1988) *Treating the Self. Elements of Clinical Psychology.* London: Guilford Press.

Woolf, V. (1927) *To the Lighthouse.* London: Hogarth.

Yalom, I.D. (1970) *The Theory and Practice of Group Psychotherapy.* New York: Basic Books.

Yalom, I.D. (1985) *The Theory and Practice of Group Psychotherapy.* (3rd Ed.) New York: Basic Books.

Subject Index

Author Index